Spirit of nature

Dedication

For my godson Zac. **David M. Bell**

Thankyou to Bec Matthews. **David**

Many thanks go to my teachers on the spiritual aspects of Traditional Chinese Medicine, especially Dr Yen (Hangzhou, China), John McDonald (Sydney and Taupo, New Zealand), Chris Madden (Sydney), and my partner, Jackie Kiddle. **James**

Disclaimer: The information and advice contained in this book is not intended to replace the services of a qualified doctor or health practitioner. Please consult your health practitioner before using any of the therapies or advice in this book. Use of any information contained herein is beyond the control of the author and the publisher who cannot be held responsible for any problems or injuries arising from its application.

Thomas C. Lothian Pty Ltd
132 Albert Road, South Melbourne, Victoria 3205
www.lothian.com.au

First published 2004

National Library of Australia
Cataloguing-in-Publication data:

Bell, David M., 1965 Dec. 2— .
Spirit of nature: the harmony of the Five Elements
—.a path to healing
ISBN 0 7344 0669 X

1. Five agents (Chinese philosophy). 2. Philosophy, Chinese. I. McNeill, James. II. Title.

113

Managing editor: Magnolia Flora
Editor: Sue Harvey
Designed by Michelle Mackintosh
Pre-press by Hell Colour Australia Pty Ltd
Printed in China by Everbest Printing

David M. Bell
with James McNeill

Spirit of nature

The harmony of the Five Elements:
a path to healing

Earth Metal Water Wood Fire

土 金 水 木 火

Lothian
BOOKS

David M. Bell

After doing basic Shiatsu training at Shiatsu Australia Educational Services, David completed a Diploma of Zen Shiatsu at Shiatsu College Aotearoa. He studied for a further three years with the School of Zen Shiatsu New Zealand, and attended master class intensives and meditation retreats with Sonia Moriceau of Healing Shiatsu.

He was privileged to also study with Robert Young of Psycho Physical Integration, and privately with Frank Quattrone, a healer and dear friend now deceased.

David lives in Melbourne, Australia, where he continues his study of oriental philosophy and divides his time between the film industry and writing. In this, his third book, he acknowledges that perhaps the greatest teacher we ever have is nature.

David wrote the main body of the text, the poems and the meditations in this book. He also took the photographs and painted the calligraphy and the Wu Xing illustrations.

www.davidbell.net.au

James McNeill

James runs a busy acupuncture practice with his partner, Jackie Kiddle, in Hawkes Bay, New Zealand. He developed an interest in Eastern philosophy from an early age. He completed a Diploma in Traditional Chinese Medicine in Sydney in 1986. This four-year course included hospital internship training in Hangzhou, China. James moved from Australia to New Zealand in 1988.

He is a past president of the New Zealand Register of Acupuncturists and a member of the Ministerial Advisory Committee for Complementary and Alternative Health. He currently divides his time between his family, the clinic and his song-writing. He has three young children.

James wrote the section 'Traditional Chinese Medicine and the Five Elements' and the Traditional Chinese Medicine section of each individual element chapter. He also contributed generally to the book in this area of expertise.

Contents

Preface

The enormity of Five Element theory and its applications is exciting; every layer peeled away reveals yet another, and the exploration is endless. The beautifully poetic and practical Five Element system is constantly evolving.

Spirit of Nature is an exploration of just that: the spirit of nature. Five Element theory doesn't exist to be revered — it exists to revere nature. We consulted acknowledged texts and compared our own training and clinical notes, but mostly the book consists of the imagery, analogy and prose we have gathered from observations of the contemporary world as seen through Five Element theory. The photographs defer to the energetic nature of their subject matter — the 'spirit' of the subject — and reflect on the interconnectedness of the macrocosm and microcosm.

Five Element theory asks that we let go and discover the calm spaciousness of being 'right here and right now'. The world around us, and within us, reveals itself not as a learned set of assertions but as the living experience of constant discovery. This is our challenge: to stop for a moment and have the wisdom to say, 'We know nothing.' This empty space allows us to have an affectionate conversation with nature — our greatest teacher — and to use the dialogue as a tool for healing.

The theory of the Five Elements

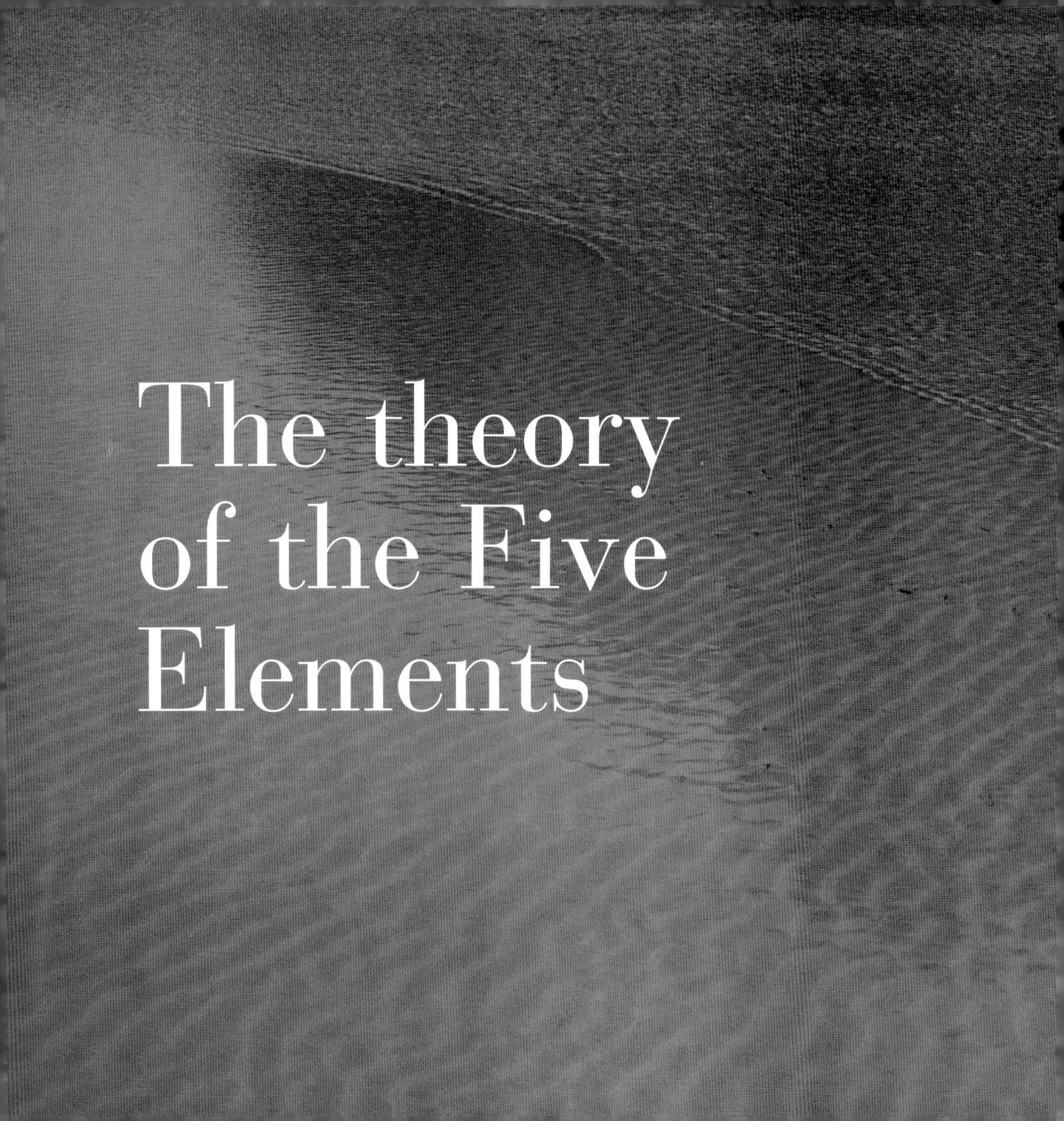

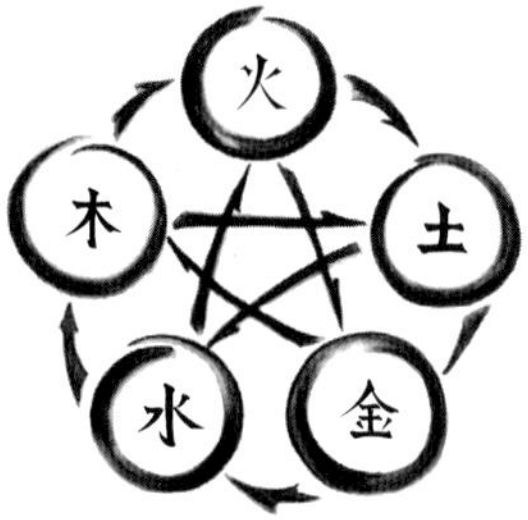

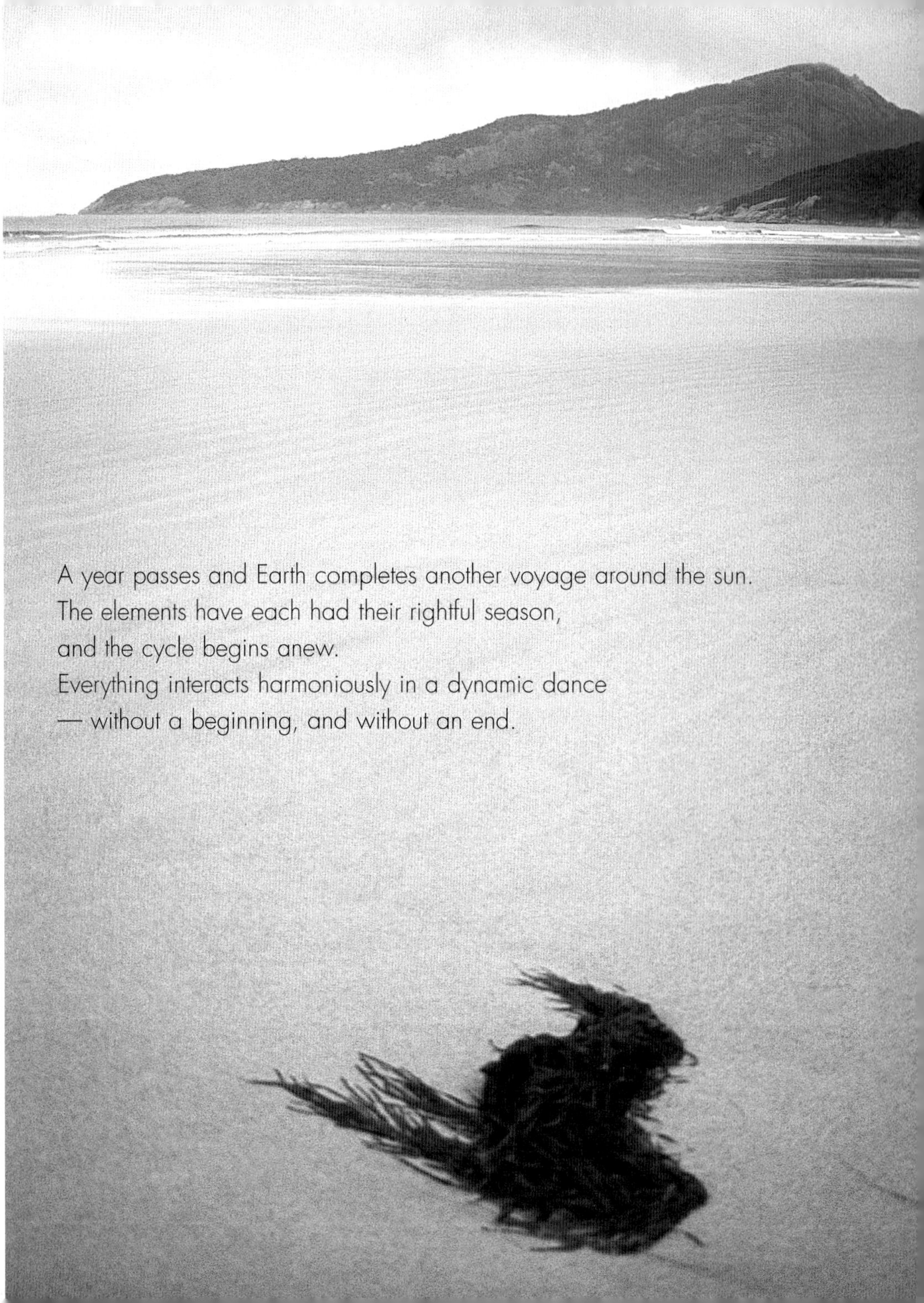

A year passes and Earth completes another voyage around the sun.
The elements have each had their rightful season,
and the cycle begins anew.
Everything interacts harmoniously in a dynamic dance
— without a beginning, and without an end.

The Five Elements: Earth, Metal, Water, Wood and Fire

We live in nature. Nature is in a constant state of flux, and movement is the lifeblood of the universe. Movement can be watched and tracked, like footprints in sand, until the emerging patterns show us a direction of travel. With these patterns we can map the journey and predict which direction the next step will take, in the same way that we map and predict the rise and fall of tides and the pattern of the seasons.

Five Element theory, which originated thousands of years ago in China, demonstrates beautifully the rhythmic flow and cyclic order of nature by observing patterns of movement. The theory maps the constant interaction of everything in the universe by signposting recognisable features and conditions. These signposts are named symbolically after phenomena found in nature — Earth, Metal, Water, Wood, Fire — and are spaced evenly throughout the known realm of creation.

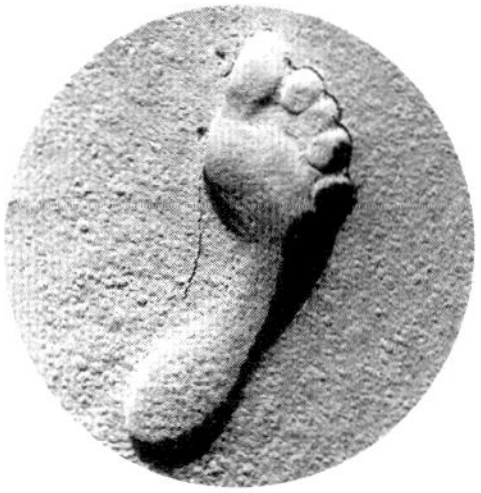

The system is beautifully encompassing. It groups together associations or correspondences that connect with, or are attributes of, each of these elements. For instance, in the temperate regions of the world we acknowledge the arrival of the Spring when the days lengthen and the trees are in blossom. The season of Spring is felt in every aspect of creation; it leaves a signature on everything it touches. We call these collective signatures Spring, but the season of Spring is not a static state or an entity in itself. In the same moment that Spring arrives it has already begun to become something else. Everything in the universe exists only in relationship to something else, and in a relationship with everything else.

A good way to explore Five Element theory is to examine each thing associated with each element until the archetypal design of the element itself becomes visible. Each of the elements can be explored with images, poetry and prose, allowing our analytical mind to rest for a moment while an intimate experience of life reveals itself.

The true nature of
a single blade of grass
reveals the workings
of the universe.

When there is an imbalance in the natural order of life, each aspect of the cycle is affected and disrupted. If the season of Spring is too weak for the blossoms to bloom, there will be no fruit, no seeds and no new trees to bear the next generation of blossom. All of the Five Elements are in constant motion and form a circle of life that has no starting point and no end. Each aspect of creation — represented by the Five Elements — must be in place for this dynamic circle of life to remain unbroken.

The Five Elements represent
the five forces of creation
in motion and explore
the nature of nature.

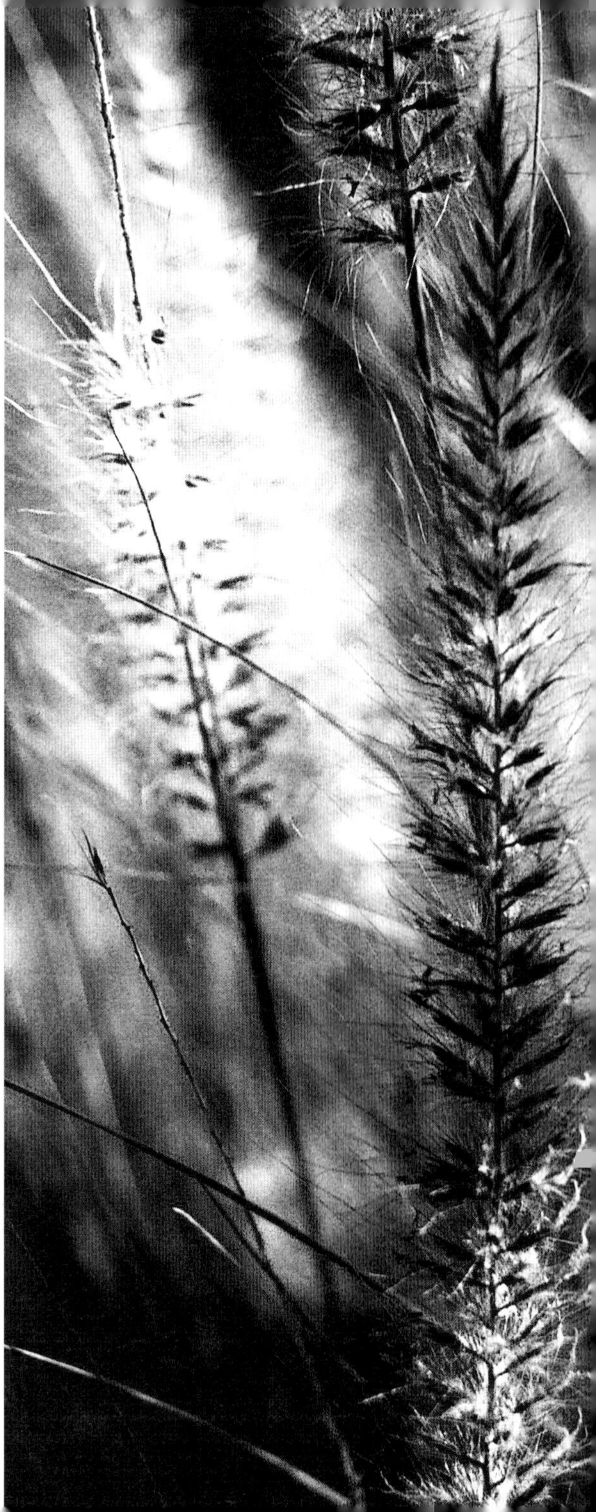

The language of Five Element theory

The Five Element theory is a living language rather than a lifeless doctrine. It is a beautiful guide to the conservation of nature and natural order. Like all languages, it evolves as we communicate the ideas and insights that we experience when we look at the world around us. By using Five Element theory we are able to converse with nature and seek the truth of our own nature. This 'truth' becomes a quest rather than a place in which to settle; Five Element theory continues to unfold and reveal new 'truths' the longer it is explored. The theory itself — while acknowledging its founders and some fundamental principles — has a life of its own.

The term 'element' describes an activity. It is a way of speaking figuratively about a phase of creation and about a set of associated occurrences for that phase. For instance, fire is used as imagery to describe a phase of creation because the properties of physical fire lend themselves well to the description. Fire doesn't refer only to the substance of flame; it also refers to the qualities of fire that are seen in things spiritual, physical and emotional. The 'Fire element' then is seen as the principal agent for bringing forth these qualities and allows us to make comparative observation with the other elements of Earth, Metal, Water and Wood. The word 'element' is readily interchangeable with 'phase' and 'agent', as well as 'force' and 'energy'.

Augmentation by practitioners over the centuries has been an important part of the development of Five Element theory. The theory is a tool that practitioners and others have used daily for thousands of years — each person wielding it in their own way. It can be honed and improved over time; people who use the theory consistently find it becomes second nature. At this point the 'tool' transcends the purely functional and its use becomes an art form.

But it is not the theory of the Five Elements that we need to revere; rather, the theory exists to revere nature. Nature teaches us. This teacher is not separate from the subject matter; the teacher and the taught are of the same body. When we look deeply into any one phenomenon of nature, including ourselves, we experience insight into the greater workings of the universe and realise that the macrocosm and the microcosm are affectionately pointing at each other. As humans we are manifestations of the greater cosmos and are never entirely separate from or unaffected by the universe around us and in us. Nature shows us how to intuitively read the signatures of the elements within ourselves and to see our role in the cyclic order of the world more clearly. Understanding these lessons is the objective of Five Element theory.

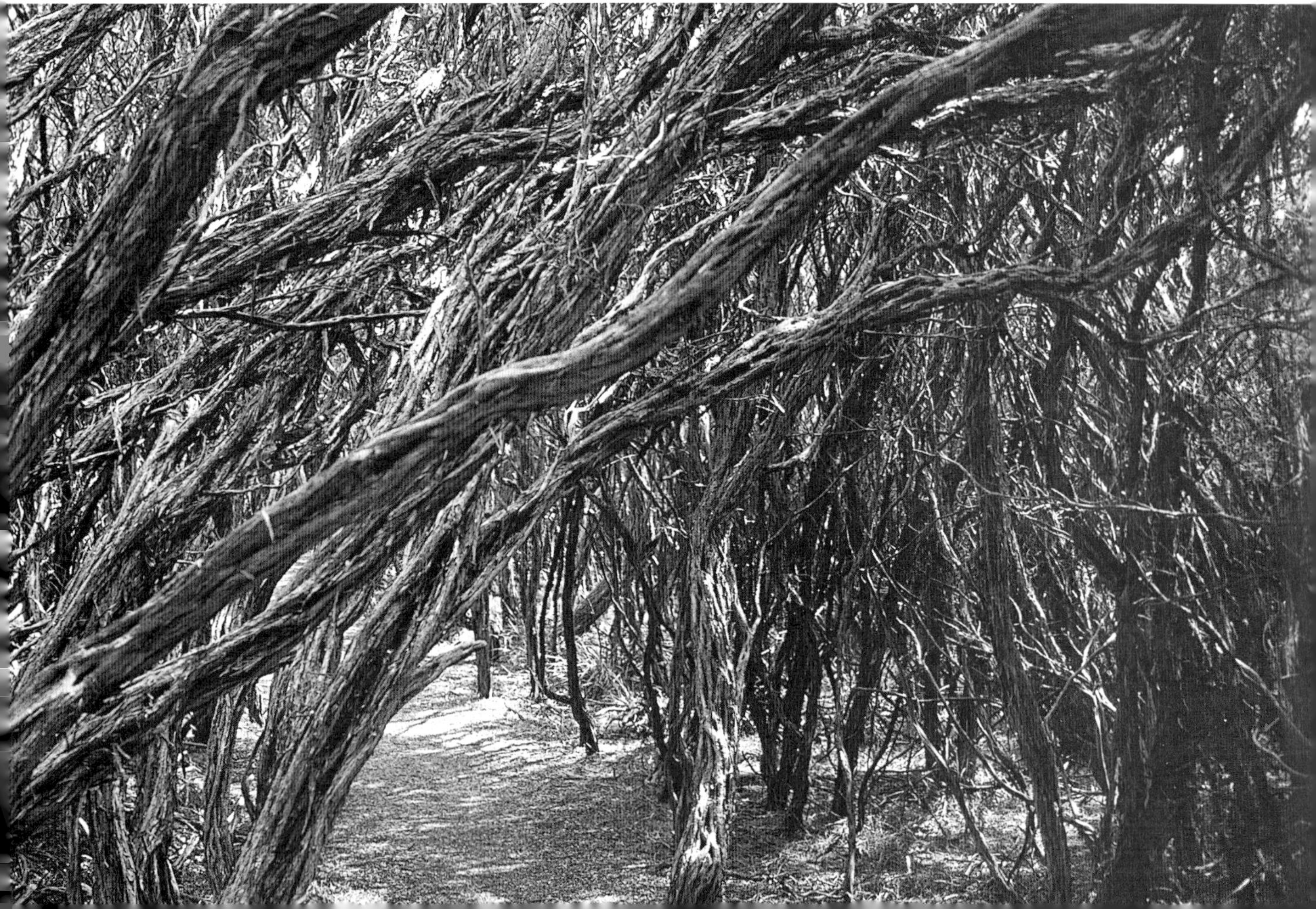

Five Element theory signposts the starting point of an amazing journey.

土 金 水 木 火

Five Element creation and destruction cycles

Where composition exists, so too does decomposition. The Five Elements complement each other in two distinct ways: each element nourishes the next element in the cycle while controlling the element adjacent. The illustration below describes the flow of these events through its two main paths of interaction — an outer 'circle' and an inner 'star'. In China this illustrated model for the Five Element system is called the Wu Xing.

The Five Elements

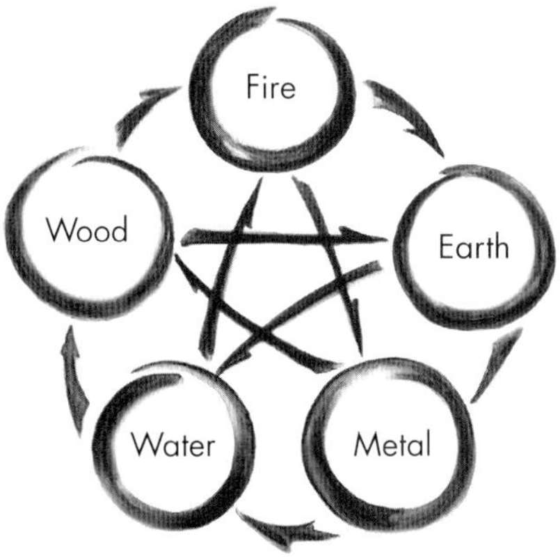

Creation (Sheng)

The first path of interaction in Five Element theory gathers together the powers of creation. This creation cycle (called Sheng in China) is concerned with generation, promotion and regeneration. Each element 'gives birth' to the next element in an act of natural continuance, and each element lends particular attributes to a harmoniously ordered system. Nothing in the construction system is held in one place and the relationship is one of giving and receiving freely in an endless cycle of creation.

Fire builds Earth
Earth bears Metal
Metal holds Water
Water nourishes Wood
Wood feeds Fire

In Traditional Chinese Medicine this relationship is referred to as 'Mother–Child'. This symbolism describes the essence of a relationship concerned with the birth and nourishment of the next generation. Sheng ensures that the beautiful fluidity of natural life-cycles is maintained and that the circle of creation remains unbroken.

The construction cycle

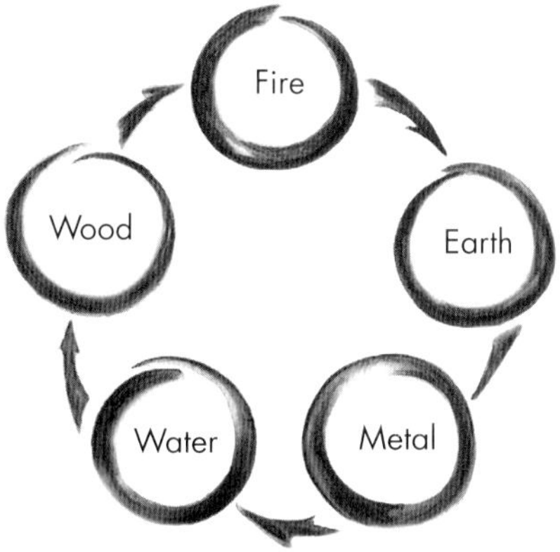

Fire cools into Earth,
which condenses into Metal,
which melts into liquid,
which takes form into Wood,
which excites into Fire …

Control (Ko)

The second main relationship of the elements is illustrated with an internal star called the 'control cycle' (Ko cycle in Chinese). In the Five Element tradition the control cycle is not seen as a negative occurrence: the elements desire harmony and so seek it by keeping each other in check with restraints and boundaries. Any excess in the natural world is detrimental to the overall ecological balance, so nature seeks patterns that are sustainable. In Five Element theory, even excessive emotions such as 'joy' (Fire) are considered undesirable and are limited in their expression by the presence of the other emotions.

The essence of this relationship is poetically rendered in the imagery of nature:

Fire melts and reduces Metal
Metal cuts and conquers Wood
Wood penetrates and draws goodness from Earth
Earth silts and inhibits the flow of Water
Water suppresses and extinguishes Fire.

The control (Ko) cycle

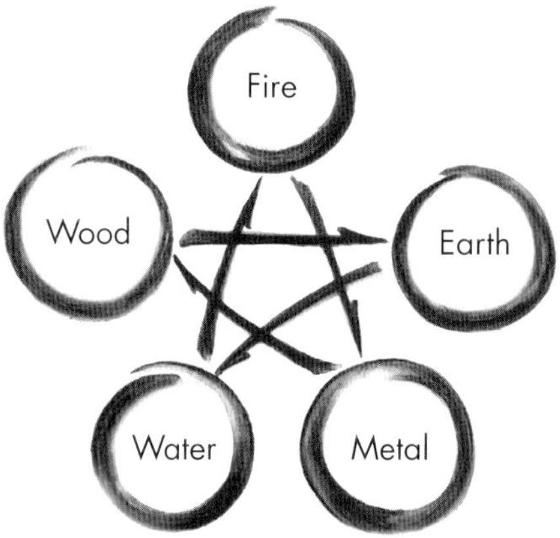

It is easy to see how the control cycle imagery might have been applied in agricultural life in Ancient China. To work with metal use fire; to cut wood use an axe; to break up the earth sow seeds or use the wooden hoe; to control the water in the rice paddy or the flooding river build earthen walls; and if the fire over which you cook gets too big, extinguish it with water.

The Ko cycle is also sometimes referred to as the 'Grandparent and child' relationship: the Grandparent keeps the grandchild in order. If this relationship is too dominant, with the Grandparent too severe, problems occur. The child might also rebel and insult the Grandparent! When this happens it is called the 'counter-control' or 'insult cycle'.

The illustration of the Ko cycle gives a good sense of the direct action that takes place in this aspect of Five Element theory. Rather than scribing a flowing circle, the Ko cycle schematic moves from one element to the next along decisive line segments — like an arm thrust outward from a body — and takes direct action!

Two work as one

Together, the two main relationships of Sheng (construct) and Ko (destruct) harmonise the interactive flow of Chi or Qi (life force) and complete the basic model for Five Element theory. Within our own bodies and within nature we find harmony in a balanced flow of Qi and find disharmony when this balance is missing. Dis-ease and dis-order can exist only in the place where balance, ease and order does not. If any of the Five Elements become too dominant or too recessive the entire order of events is affected.

The Wu Xing illustrations teach of the Five Elements by providing us with tools for identifying and preventing the causes of disorder. These tools are used as an underlying philosophy in many arts and therapies: Traditional Chinese Medicine (including acupuncture, herbs, exercises, acupressure massage and moxibustion), Shiatsu, Feng Shui, many martial arts, Traditional Korean Medicine, Traditional Japanese Medicine, Chinese Astrology and Qi Gong. The application of Five Element theory demonstrates great flexibility and has been assimilated into healing practices all over the world.

Associations of the elements

In space, when we look at the unnumbered stars, we divide what we see into named clusters so we can share an understanding of grouped identities within the enormity of the universe. Every named group is only a part of a still larger group with no known finality.

Five Element theory is a cosmology that groups together expressions of life into five named clusters — Earth, Metal, Water, Wood, Fire. Each element has its own associated season, organs, smell, taste, direction, colour, time of day and countless other qualities and forms of expression. Some of these associations are easily accepted with our logical minds and stem directly from the imagery of nature:

The colour of Fire is red.
The season for Fire is summer.
The emotion for Fire is joy.

Other associations derive from a more intuitive understanding of the natural world and have developed over thousands of years of observation, experience and insight. The origins of these associations are not as obvious at a glance and begin to make delightful sense when the Five Element theory becomes better known.

The sense organ associated with the Wood element is the eyes.
The sound associated with the Metal element is weeping.
The taste associated with the Earth element is sweet.

No association is a stand-alone fact. The associations are part of an understanding of the Dao: everything is a collection of many other things, and is a part of something greater. Together, the associations or tendencies create an 'identity' for each element and 'locate' each element so we can reference it. This is how we can philosophically navigate the vastness of heaven and earth and watch the interplay of the forces of creation. In so doing we see the relationship and correlation between humans and all other aspects of nature.

The basic classification of phenomena according to the Five Elements is depicted in the table on page 25.

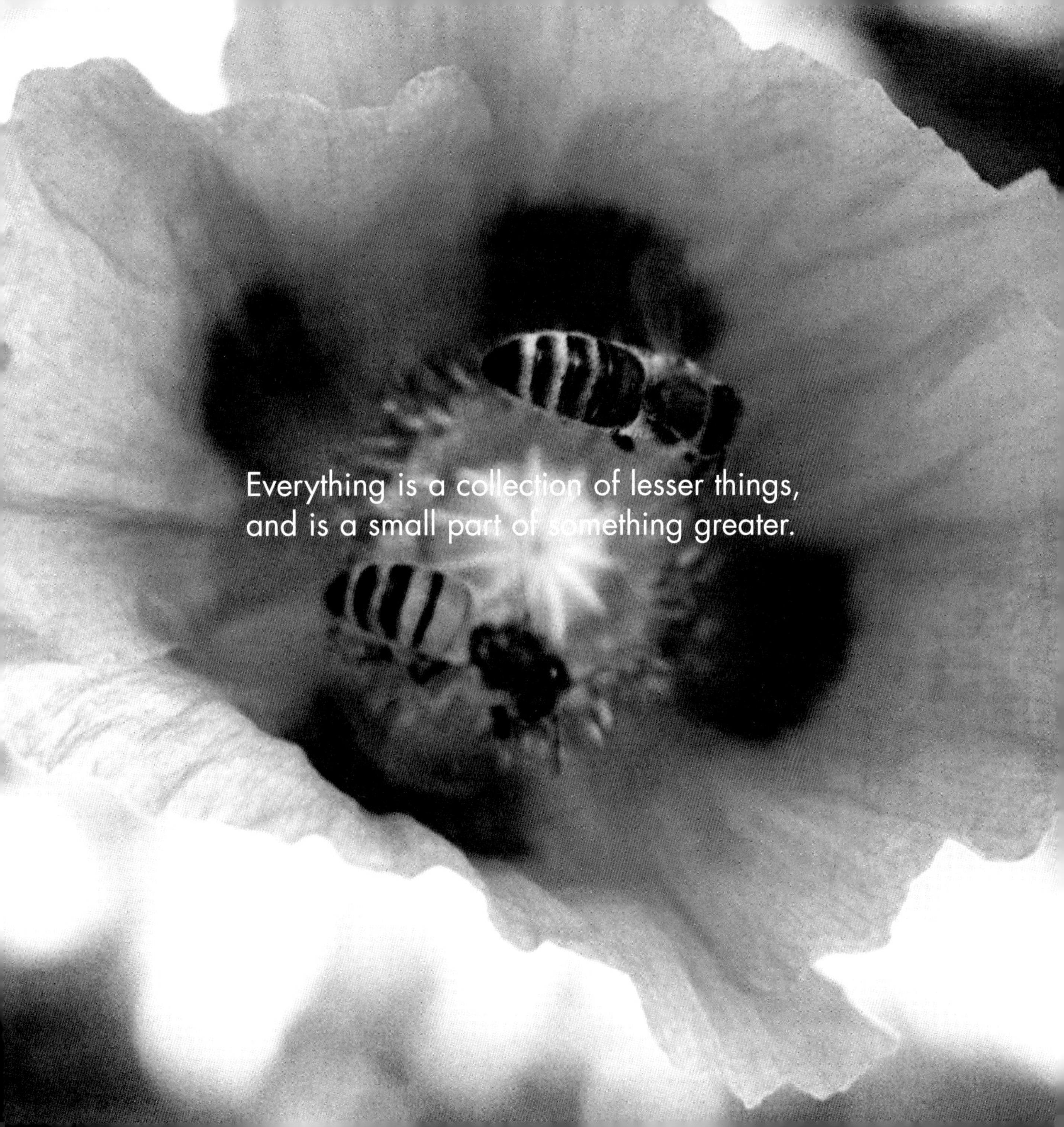

Everything is a collection of lesser things,
and is a small part of something greater.

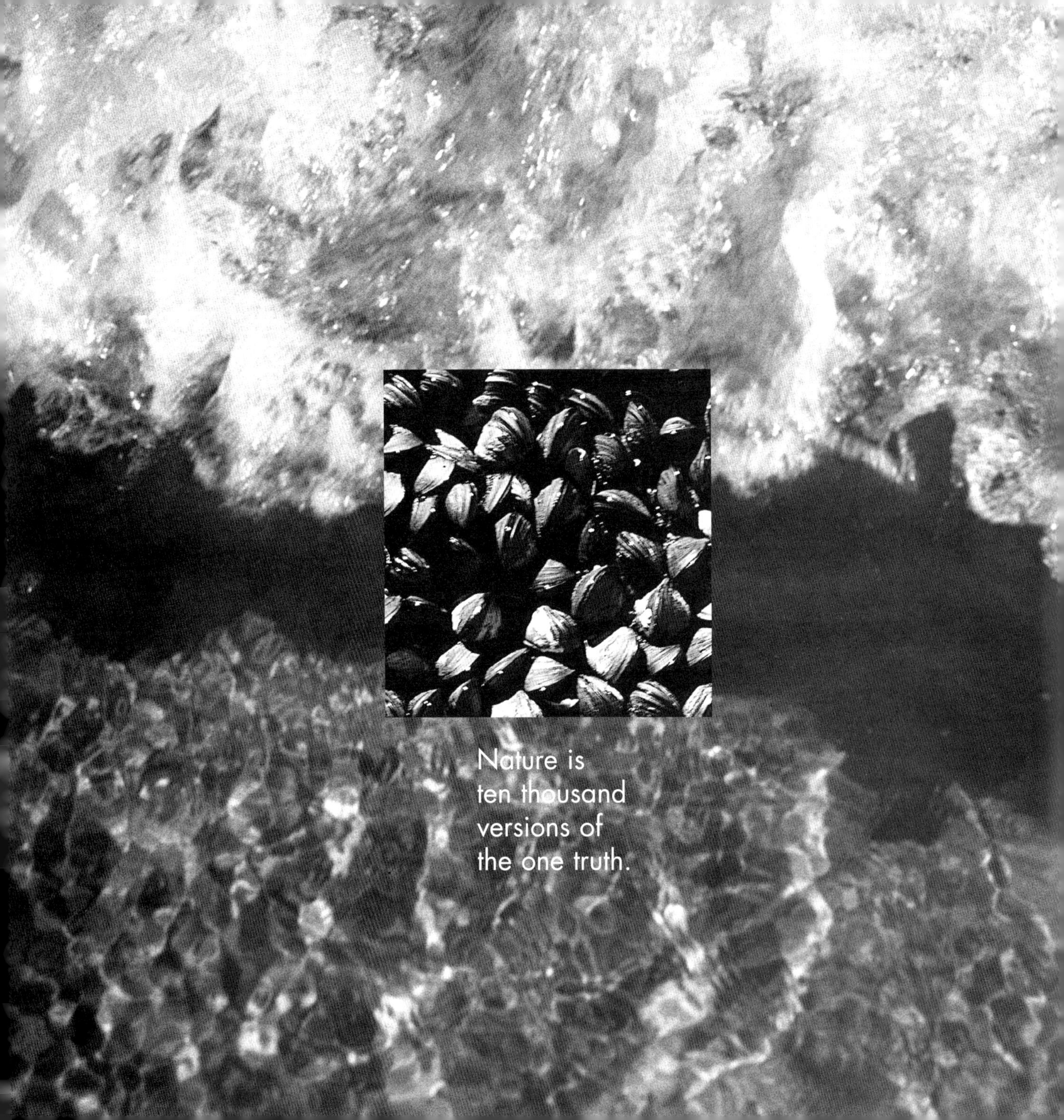

Nature is
ten thousand
versions of
the one truth.

Basic classification of phenomena according to the Five Elements

Phenomena	Earth	Metal	Water	Wood	Fire
Yang organ	Stomach	Large intestine	Bladder	Gall bladder	Small intestine
Yin organ	Spleen	Lung	Kidney	Liver	Heart
Emotion	Sympathy	Grief	Fear	Anger	Joy
Expression	Singing	Weeping	Groaning	Shouting	Laughing
Body tissue	Muscle (flesh)	Hair and skin	Bone	Tendons	Vessels (blood)
Sense organ	Mouth	Nose	Ears	Eyes	Tongue
Season	Late summer	Autumn	Winter	Spring	Summer
Colour	Yellow	White	Black	Green	Red
Orientation	Centre	West	North	East	South
Climate (adverse)	Damp (humidity)	Dryness	Cold	Wind	Heat
Taste	Sweet	Pungent	Salty	Sour	Bitter

Adapted primarily from *The Essentials of Chinese Acupuncture*, Foreign Languages Press, Beijing, China, 1980.

The ingredients of Five Element theory

The phenomena of Dao, Qi, and Yin and Yang are not separate from the Five Element theory. They are part of the same story.

To understand Five Element theory we need to understand some of the tenets of Chinese philosophy. The Dao, Yin–Yang theory and Qi are all vital aspects of the bigger picture that incorporates Five Element theory.

The Dao (way of the universe) is the eternal one thing, with no separate identity, that contains all things.

Qi exists within the Dao and is the pure ingredient of all life — the life force.

Yin and Yang are the dynamic complementary 'divisions' of the life force.

The Five Elements are the manifestations of the life force in constant motion.

The Dao

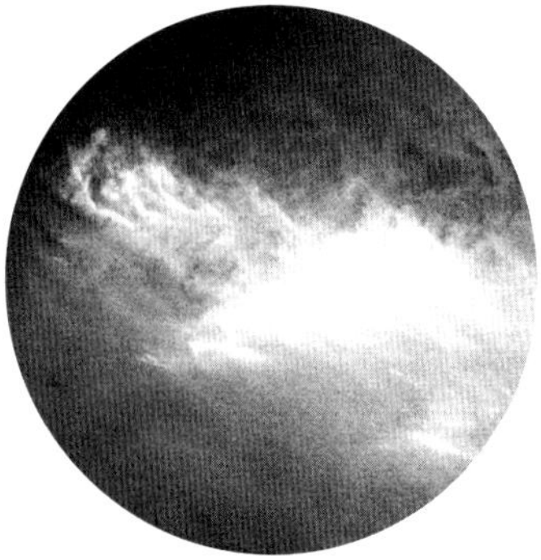

Although it creates the universe,
it is not separate.
Although we name it,
we have not found it.

Part of the joy of appreciating the Dao is to accept that we can never fully understand it with thought processes alone. Acceptance of mystery is an important part of traditional Chinese philosophy generally: it allows delight in phenomena beyond our comprehension.

The Dao does nothing,
and still everything is done.
The Dao creates all things,
but does not claim them.

While everything is an aspect of the Dao, the Dao has no separate identity. The Dao is simply, and profoundly, the true nature of nature that is perpetually becoming itself. The Five Elements are sub-grouped aspects of the Dao and are dynamic agents of the Dao in motion.

The Dao — being the source of all Qi — gives possibility to the five agents of essence that are the creators of all life.

The Dao is often approached with imagery, poetry and anecdote, and is more likely to 'show up' when we are not trying to point straight at it. The Dao has a lovely way of being glimpsed just before disappearing from our view altogether. Meditation can enhance a sense of oneness with the Dao by stilling our thoughts and creating a space of 'no mind': a space of consciousness in the absence of thoughts.

Collectively, every single thing in the universe forms the 'ultimate reality' of the Dao; it is the ear that hears as well as what is heard. But the Dao remains as more than the sum total of its parts; all phenomena are merely constituents of the Dao. The Dao is the container that holds all things without holding a form of its own.

The Dao has sometimes been deified through the image of a legendary character called Lao Tzu ('Great Master'), the credited author of the *Dao Te Ching*, a Chinese text from the fourth century BCE. It remains uncertain whether Lao Tzu was one person or a pseudonym for the work of many. The *Dao Te Ching* is a beautiful text and a founding work in any discussion of the Dao. It has inspired many of the poems in this book.

The Daoist sages seek the nature of the Dao — the Way. They live with the knowledge that they themselves are a visible manifestation of the Dao, as is the world, but that the Dao is not limited to a collection of things visible or physical. In the spirit of the Dao, the creator and creation find no separation, and worship has no singular focus.

Dao

All of heaven and earth, things known and unknown, issue from the One.
Light and dark separate their names and live in their mother's realm.
The Dao cannot be defined by motion or form and has no end.
There is no measure, no quantity, and no one true name.
Myriad nature abides the law and exists together.
All life exists only because of its neighbour.
The things inherent to this universe
live because of interaction.
There is no separation
within the One,
or of the
One.

Qi is everything
except something in itself.
Qi is what it does,
not what it is.

Qi: the underlying force

Qi can be described in many ways: life force, vital essence, universal energy, cosmic breath, life's spirit. However, Qi is not abstract and some of these terms suggest something distant or distinct from our everyday life. Qi is the force that animates the invisible into the visible; it courses through all that we call 'alive', and even what we think of as inorganic. In many Asian countries, Qi is discussed in everyday language and is not mystified.

Qi is like a vibration that instigates the existence of matter and the event of the Five Elements. Qi is the pre-emptive essence of matter — the underlying force — and is the basic ingredient of matter itself. Movement and Qi are inseparable, just as Qi and the Five Elements are inseparable; Qi is the verb of life. It can be channelled, summoned, extended forth and used in everyday contexts.

Qi is recognisable by what it becomes and by the movement it initiates. Five Element theory describes the manifestations and movements of Qi by using imagery from known substances in the natural world. The result is a map of the interplay of Qi as it flows throughout nature.

Qi in human beings

Traditional Chinese Medicine recognises three basic primary sources of Qi in the human body:

Inherited (prenatal) Qi is the Qi we receive from our parents, with the particular assistance of the Water element.

Air Qi is the Qi we gather from the air through respiration, with the particular assistance of the Metal element.

Food Qi is the Qi we transform from ingested matter, with the particular assistance of the Earth element.

Most traditional Asian medical practices work closely with Qi, looking at the availability of Qi in the patient, its distribution and its strength. Many martial arts also use knowledge of Qi to move with strength and to unify body, mind and spirit. The Chinese art of Tai Chi is a good example and the name reveals the intention: *tai* means supreme or great, *chi* is Qi. In the combative styles the student learns that using Qi is superior to using muscular strength alone, and that a small person with 'good Qi' can easily overcome a larger person who has little. Qi is seen as boundless; it is the force that spins the heavenly planets. With breath exercises, physical training and visualisation it can be encouraged to flow in the body.

Some other practices and therapies that understand and encourage stimulation of Qi are Do-ín, Qi Gong, Aikido, Shiatsu, Daoist Yoga, Reiki, Makaho and acupuncture.

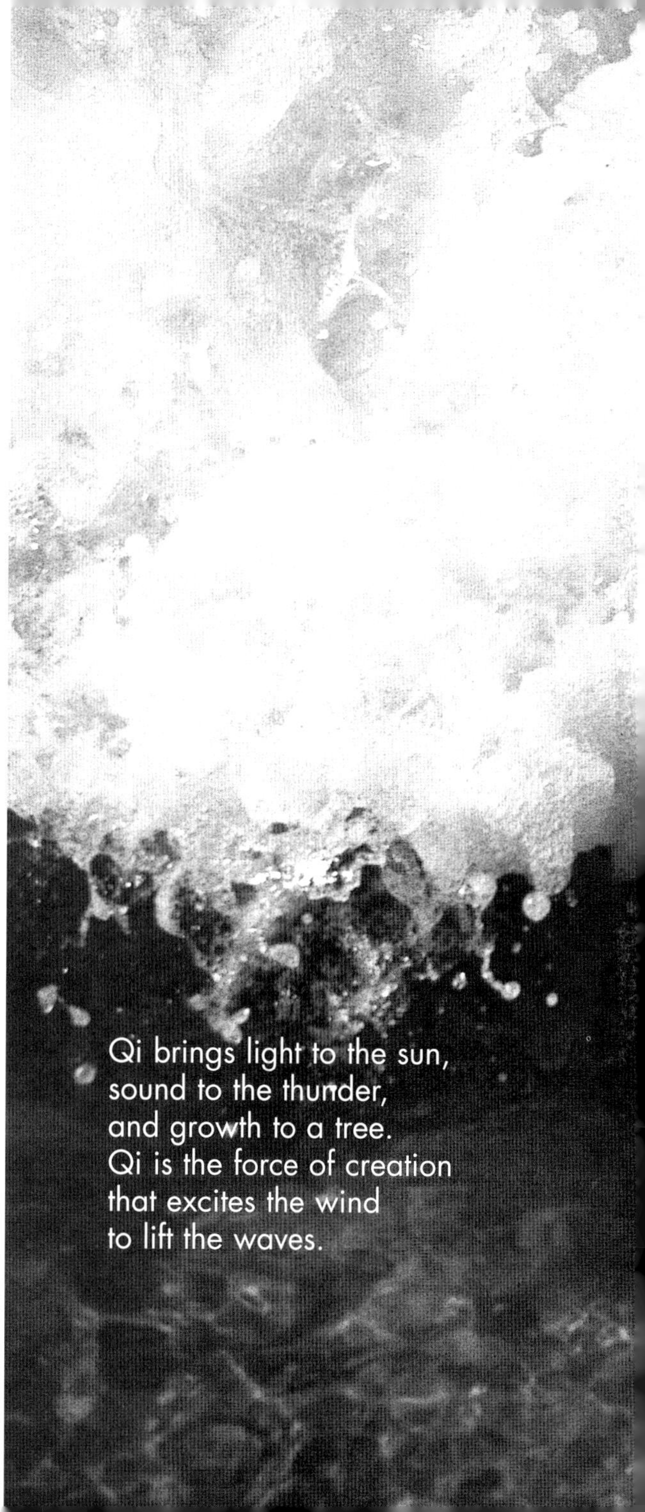
Qi brings light to the sun,
sound to the thunder,
and growth to a tree.
Qi is the force of creation
that excites the wind
to lift the waves.

Yin–Yang

The tension between opposites at the point where they meet is a place of dynamic harmony.

Traditional Chinese Medicine and other modalities that use Five Element theory emphasise the balancing of Yin and Yang within the elements. Yin and Yang are names given to describe two polarities that operate together within every aspect of creation; each of the five elements in nature contains both Yin and Yang qualities. For example, each element has Yin organs and Yang organs, Yin foods and Yang foods, 'positive' emotions and 'negative' emotions. Yin and Yang make each other and inevitably are each other; they are partners in an inseparable relationship — there can be no 'front' without the existence of a 'back'.

The Yin–Yang theory is a way of watching energetic change in the world so we can compare what we observe. An object or manifestation might be 'more Yang' than another or 'more Yin' than it was before. We can watch the cause and effect of energetic exchange and see that all aspects of life are only ever relative to other aspects. Neither state of Yin or Yang exists independently and a definitive comparison between the two can never be drawn. Although they rise and fall, vying for space, they cannot consume each other because ultimately they already contain each other.

Yin becomes Yang, Yang becomes Yin.
They are not one, nor are they two.

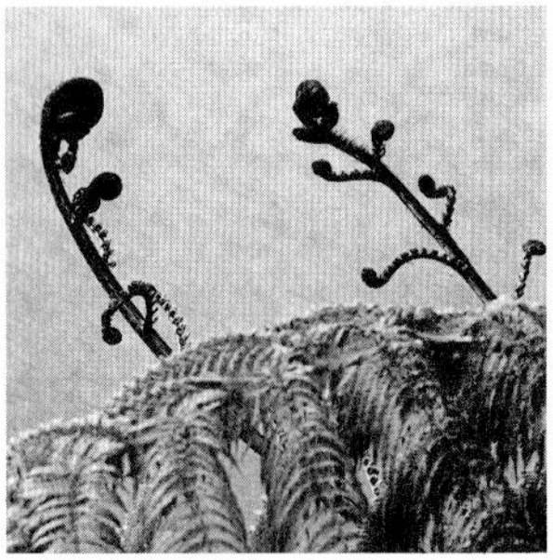

Asian philosophy doesn't view Yin or Yang as good or bad when in their natural state of balance. Yin and Yang are at once complementary and antagonistic towards each other and thereby provide the necessary tension that exists within and between all aspects of creation. Yin–Yang theory is not abstract; it is born of practical observation of our natural world and is a philosophy used to describe and seek balance. Imagine the fertile plains of Ancient China; imagine Yang being the sun and Yin the rain. Together these are 'opposites' in a co-operative union: too much sun causes a drought and too much rain a devastating flood. The healthy combination brings harmony to the land.

The symbol of Yin and Yang

The line where Yin and Yang meet within the symbol is depicted as a wave running though a sphere. This illustrates the dynamic of constant advance and retreat of yin energy and yang energy. The sphere itself is the symbol of unity and balance.

Within the shady area assigned to Yin there is a little circle of Yang, and within the sunny area assigned to Yang there is a little circle of Yin. This illustrates that there are no absolutes in nature. Everything exists as relative to something else. What is called Yang may be called Yin in relation to something else and everything that is Yin or Yang can be further broken down into still more Yin and Yang.

The Yin–Yang symbol suggests motion (while suggesting calm) and depicts opposites in harmonious union. It has been used to represent many ideologies. Sometimes it is referred to as the Tai Chi, sometimes as the Daoist symbol. In Japan it is called In and Yo.

The relative tendencies attributed to Yin and Yang are provided in the table on page 35.

Traditional Chinese Medicine and the Five Elements

Medicine or Art?

The Five Element system has remained at the core of Traditional Chinese Medicine throughout China's long recorded history and is used as a potent weapon against disease. An understanding of 'universalism', shared with Daoist and Confucian philosophies, is fundamental to Traditional Chinese Medicine — a system of health care that acknowledges the interconnectedness of all things.

Acupuncture and Chinese herbal medicine are the most well known treatments in Traditional Chinese Medicine, but many practices share similar understandings of the Five Elements. Countries such as Korea and Japan have used the philosophies to develop their own valued and diverse treatments.

Buddhism (especially the Mahayana tradition) played an important role in introducing the Five Element theory into other countries in Asia: the Buddhist texts carried by monks from China taught people to read Chinese calligraphy. Consequently, people were also able to study the philosophical tenets of pre-Buddhist Chinese culture and read texts regarding Confucianism, Daoism, Yin–Yang theory, Five Element theory and other aspects of Traditional Chinese Medicine.

The introduction of Western medical viewpoints into Traditional Chinese Medicine — some accepted, some disputed — is also part of a never-ending metamorphosis. Because the philosophies behind Traditional Chinese Medicine seek to understand the ever-changing nature of the universe, we are challenged to walk a path of constant discovery. Traditional Chinese Medicine, while maintaining distinct and pure fundamental principles and origins, accommodates the many and ever-changing environments in which it is practised.

Points: the notes of the song

Along the channels there are 365 main points and many other extra points that influence the state of Yin and Yang in the body. An acupuncture point is like a cave or hollow and the intention of the therapist is to call upon the healing qualities that live within the point. These are points that have known effects to treat different imbalances. If the channels are like the strings of the instrument then the points are those places where a note can be altered. How much one of our notes is flat or sharp is compared to the whole chord. This determines the nature of adjustment to a point, whether it be using acupuncture, massage or some other treatment.

The channels and organs of the Five Elements

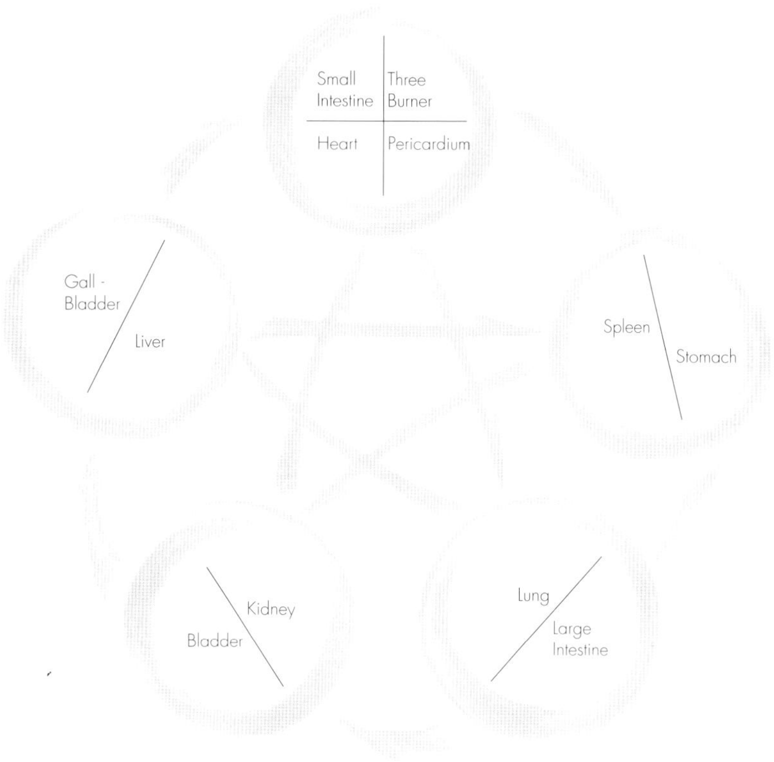

The origins of the channels and points

How the channels and points came to be perceived in the first place is one of the greatest mysteries of Traditional Chinese Medicine. There are many theories ranging from the obvious to the esoteric.

The more esoteric viewpoint is that these channels and points were intuited by minds trained to see the whole through the partial and the universal through the individual. Treatment methods were shared, recorded, refined and then tested for their effect. It is probable that the theory of the channels and the points developed through a combination of philosophical reasoning, intuitive insight, and careful observation of what was clinically useful.

Traditional Chinese Medicine disciplines the mind of the therapist to work intuitively with the Five Element system in understanding and classifying sets of information that present like so many flavours and colours. The resulting multi-dimensional picture emphasises that the whole being is so much more than just the sum of its parts.

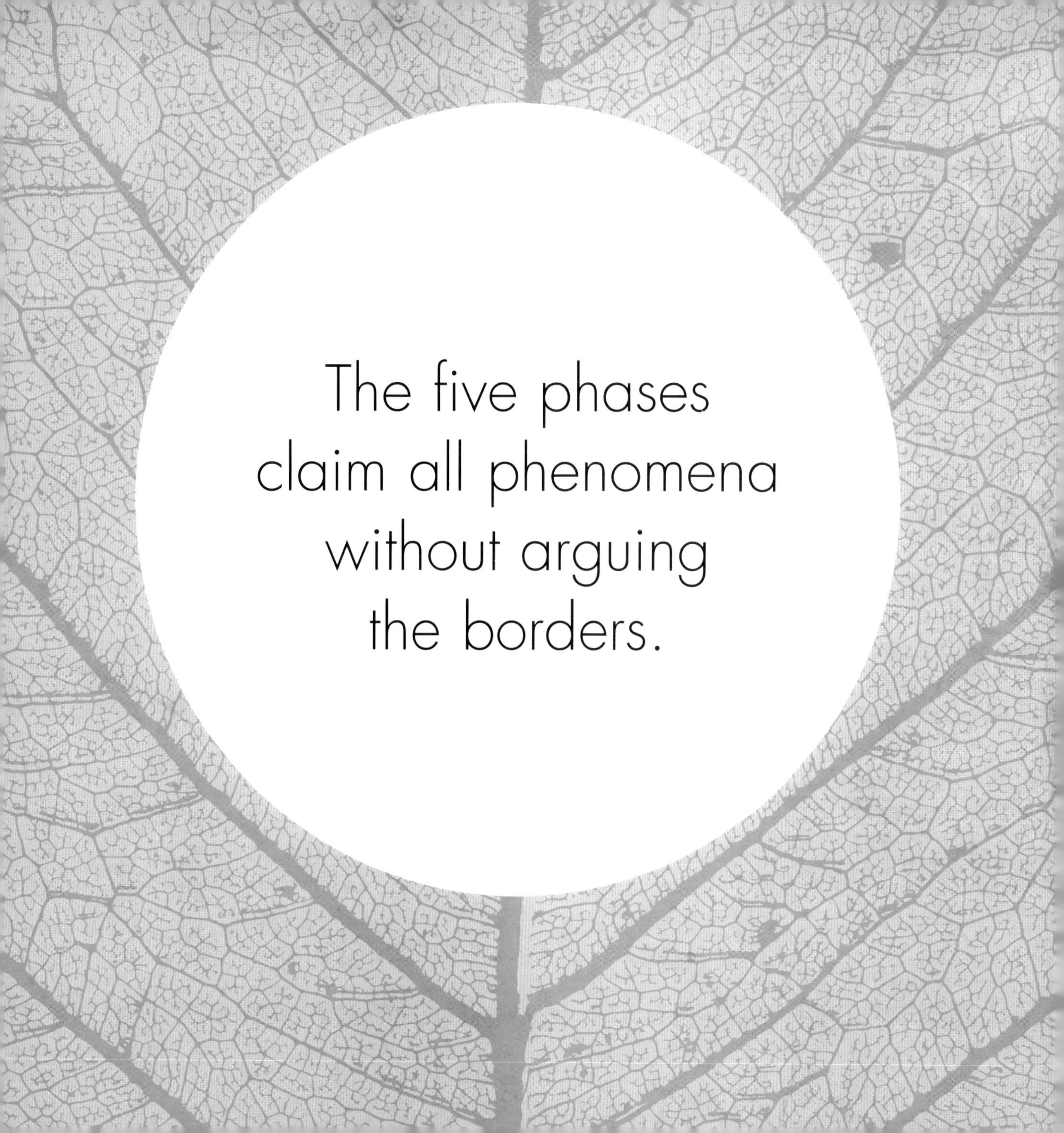

The five phases
claim all phenomena
without arguing
the borders.

Meditating on the Five Elements

Contemplating the elements in nature is a meditation in itself. Whether we use the Chinese Five Element system, or the Ayurvedic or the Greek system, we engage a tool that aids deep contemplation of the natural world. This contemplation gives focus to our minds and engenders insight.

Meditation can be active. Zen practitioners, for example, have long used forms of art and expression to focus the mind and defer to the genius of nature. These arts are in fact meditations on the spirit of nature. For instance, Zen paintings are not faithful renditions of what the eye sees; they are expressions of a spiritual practice that seeks the essential true nature and realisation of the world, and ultimately the realisation of 'self' — an objective of meditation. The ink and the empty space in a sumi-e painting work together to reveal the energetic quality and archetypal design of both the subject and the artist.

Poetry, too, has a similar ability to capture the innate nature of an unsullied moment of pure expression — the spirit of an occasion. Poetry is often concerned with the substance of the subject rather than the representation of it, and the true nature of the topic lends itself to the words with powerful delicacy. Music too can be the language of nature and become a form of meditation.

Meditation practice is concerned with the philosophy of healing and the maintenance of peaceful harmony in the world. In practices such as *zazen* (sitting meditation in the Zen tradition — from Chinese *T'so Ch'an*) using our breath as a focus in meditation brings awareness and stills the mind. In practice we cease to wander in our thoughts between the past and the future, and we begin to experience the calm nature of living mindfully. Mindfulness refers to being wholly present in the moment that is now. To be mindful is to be absolutely and calmly awake to the contemporary nature of life: 'here' rather than on the way to 'there'; 'being' instead of 'doing'. When we achieve stillness in our mind our body begins to heal itself and the world immediately around us benefits from a peaceful presence.

Meditation brings acceptance of the moment, and acceptance brings compassion. By accepting where we are instead of where we want to be, we begin to heal and to shine a light on the darkness in our life and the lives of others. Positive changes start to occur. Pain, both physical and emotional, is as much a part of our life as the things that make us happy. To avoid darkness can be exhausting and to explore darkness without a light is frightening. Being mindful of everything that arises in our life allows us to look at events in our life, as they occur, with a clear mind and a compassionate heart. Then we are able to delight in the spirit of nature and discover qualities of our own nature.

The Five Elements offer a beautiful focus for our meditations.
To contemplate deeply the workings of the cosmos and our role in the natural world is an act of love.

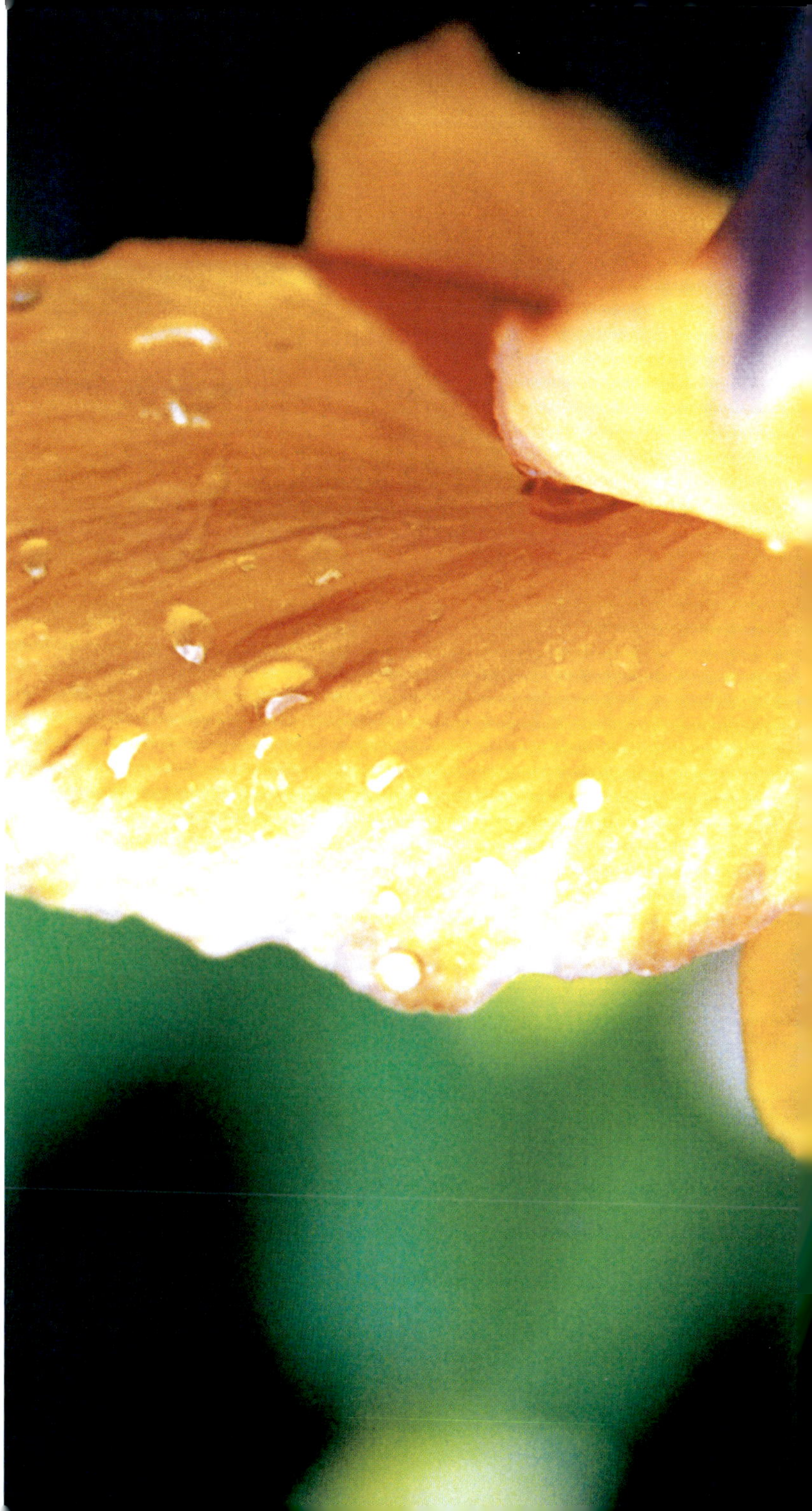

土 金 水 木 火 The Five Elements

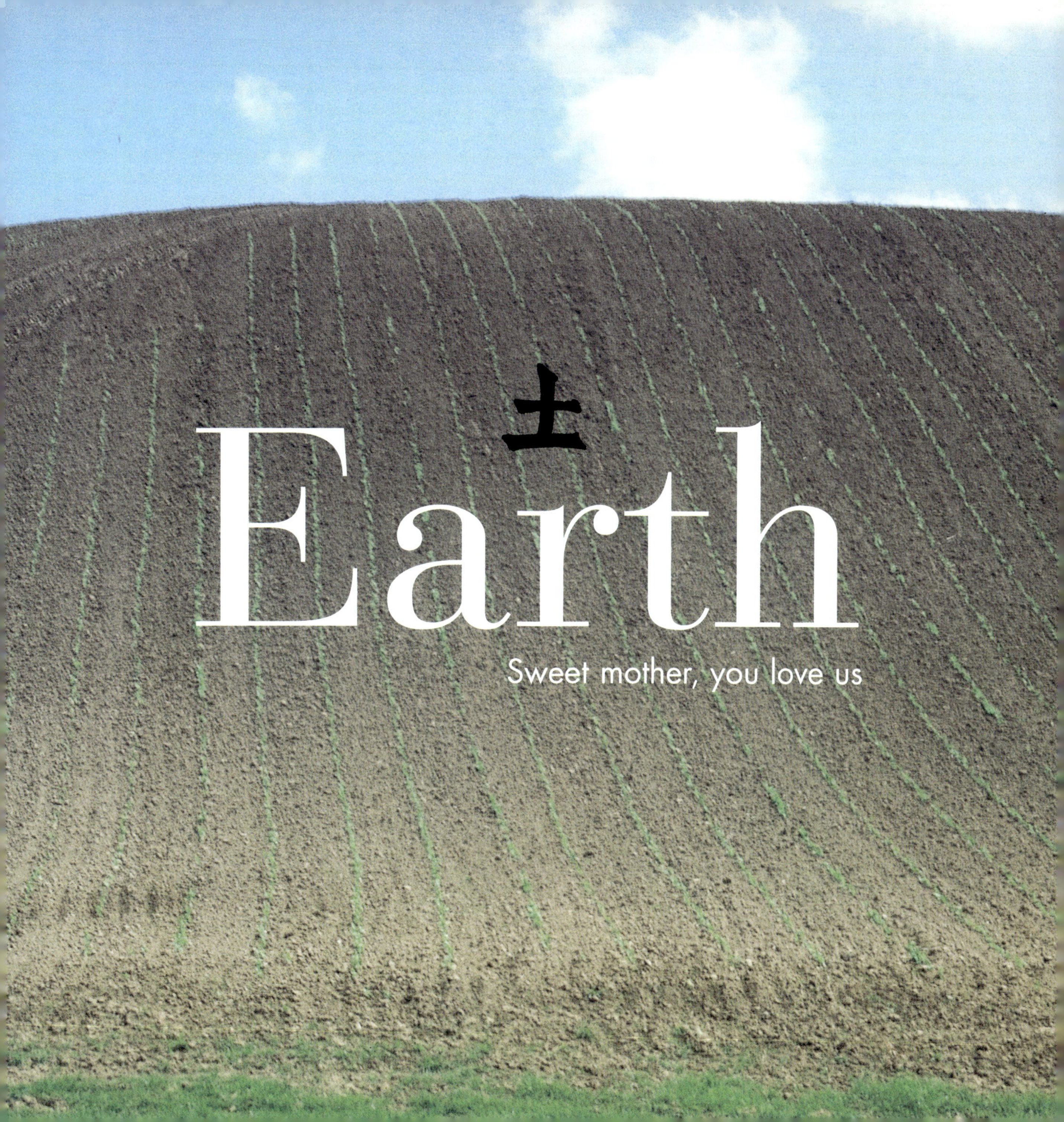
土
Earth
Sweet mother, you love us

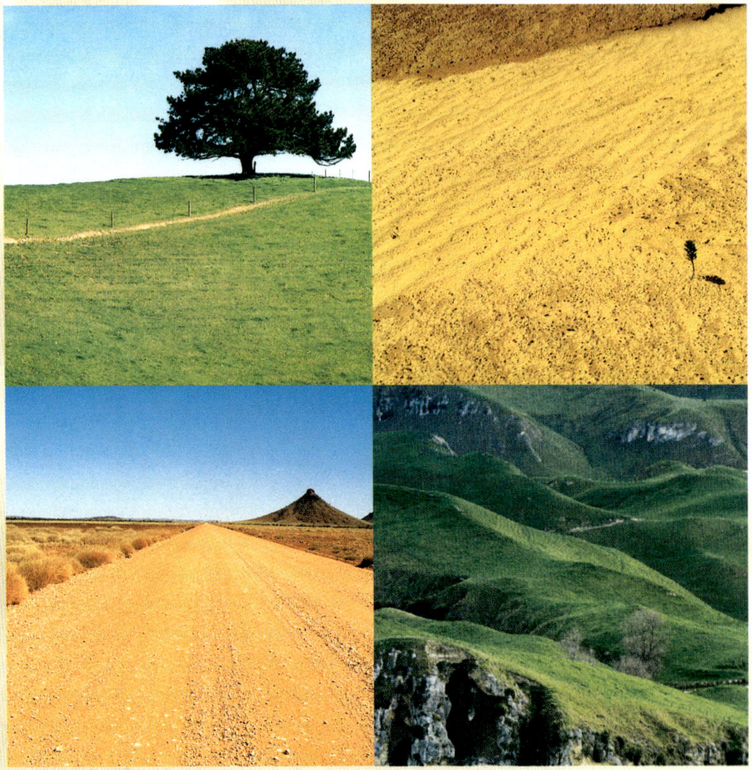

Earth

Come to me,
and these arms will enfold you.
This is your home — I am your mother.
All things gather here
to share the most simple of pleasures;
to gather food,
to be nurtured.

I am at your centre — sweet and fragrant,
the embodiment of compassion
and transformation.
I am the fertile womb
and the suckled breast;
my soil is moist and rich,
my season late and overripe.

My sands carry stories of the spirit
and of inner worlds.
I am your form and flesh,
your mouth,
your birth,
the ground beneath your feet.

Sing to me — I give you an abundant gift.
I am the foundation of this life,
I am the manifestation
of Earth.

Traditional Chinese Earth element associations:

Late summer, yellow, humidity, muscle and flesh, the mouth, singing, sympathy and compassion, the spleen, the stomach, the centre, sweet flavours.

The Earth element expressed in nature

The creative power of the Earth element expresses itself in the natural world primarily as soil. The energetic activity known as the 'Earth element' takes the physical forms of soil and sand; it is in soil that we see the productive nature of this element. Soil is alive! A handful of soil has richness, texture and a smell that speaks to our hearts of the sweet sensuality of life. The living energy of the Earth element provides the very ground beneath our feet — the building block and backbone of all that sustains our earthly existence.

Food is the 'fruit of the earth' expressed in the abundance of flora, and the Earth element is seen as the primary provider in the elemental interplay that creates food. The soil that provides this food is in a constant state of recycling as it both gives and receives of itself. It is replenished by ageing trees and rotting fruit while it simultaneously nurtures the new sapling and the growth of fresh food. Five Element theory identifies the Earth element as the agent of ripening and rotting.

Fecundity and fertility are strong features of the Earth element's qualities both within humans and within the natural world. In the absence of these qualities soil is described as barren or infertile — the imagery reflects the fact that the Earth element is the central provider of physical life. A gardener understands, as did the Ancient Chinese, that the soil must be nurtured if it is to remain productive and continue to bear provisions for the future generations.

As we move away from the river flats and the green hills, the yellow sands of the desert bring a feeling of age and peace to our hearts. Many of the world's great religions come from these lands of sand, which have been aged by sun and wind for thousands of years. At once harsh and fragile, the desert is the great matured body of the Earth now unconcerned with physical fertility, and is a place of meditative reflection that is rich with spiritual fertility.

This is a land free of distractions; it allows us to perceive of inner worlds and to see that the outer world can reveal itself to us in the smallest of details, even in a simple play of light. People who live and travel by the moods of the desert revere the beauty of the desert's power and of the mother — the Earth. Contemplation and meditation are strong qualities of the traditional Earth element.

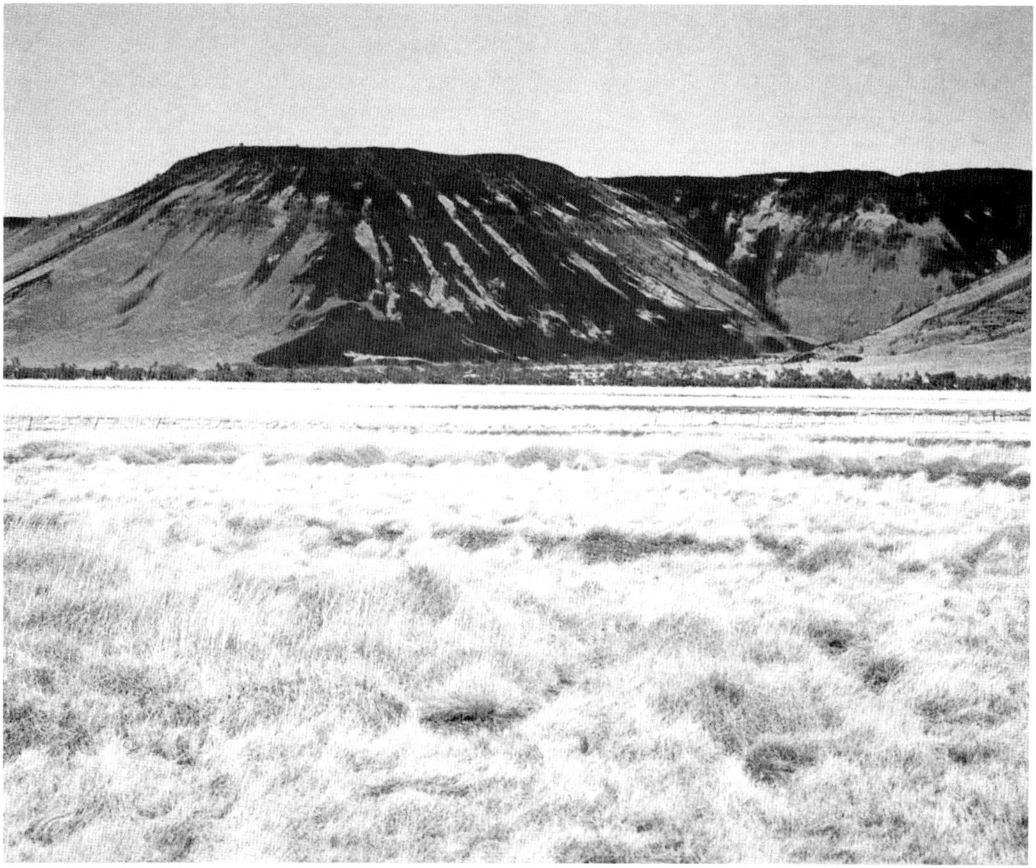

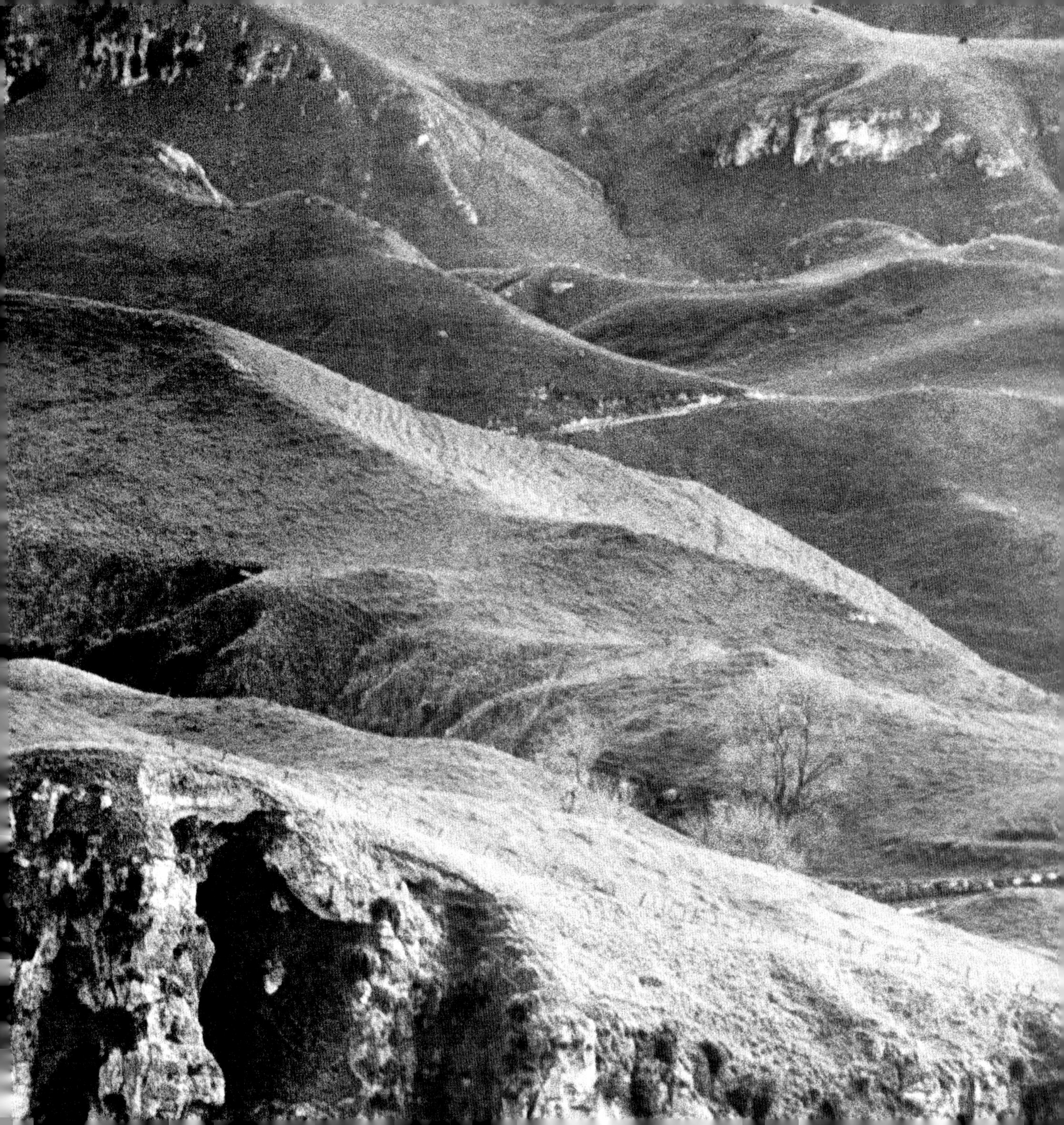

As 'earthlings' we naturally revere our abode, having no other. We feel displaced only when we have ceased to understand our place in the realm of phenomena or when we have forgotten the gifts of the mother. To be 'earthy' is to be connected with the natural world and to be a person who knows strongly of their own existence, without affectation.

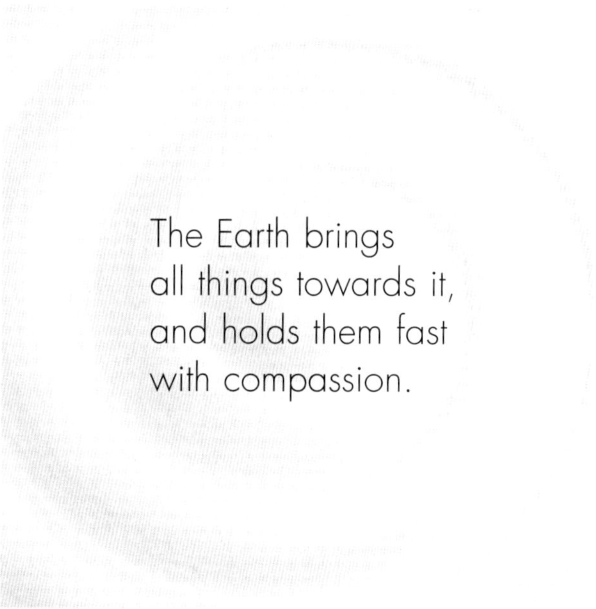

The Earth brings
all things towards it,
and holds them fast
with compassion.

Earth energy makes us feel grounded. A grounded person feels at home on this planet and is able to deal clearly with the everyday problems that arise, as they arise. But a person can stand their ground too firmly and people with strong Earth element energy need to watch for dogmatism.

The builder of form

Traditionally, the Earth element is the agent for the centralisation of all things of the world. The energetic intention — or direction — that Earth energy creates is 'downwards' or centralising. Earth absorbs and reunites the physical forces of creation in order to enrich itself and grow new life forms. The Earth element holds together the Qi that builds these physical forms and facilitates the assimilation of energy that mobile creatures need in order to move. Earth is the platform for physical experience — the body of existence. It carries the memory and remains of the myriad life forms that have come before.

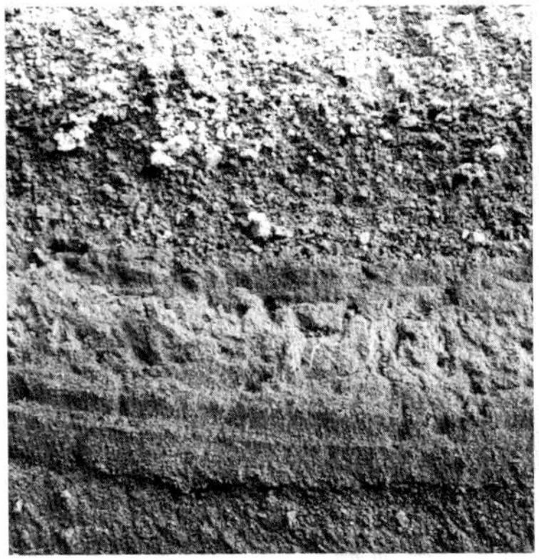

The Earth element provides the common ground for the interaction of all the elements, like a canvas rich in possibilities for the untold expressions of life. Without Earth's energy we are without body, and remain as unworldly entities. The elements need a home in which to experience their existence, and so do we. That home is Earth.

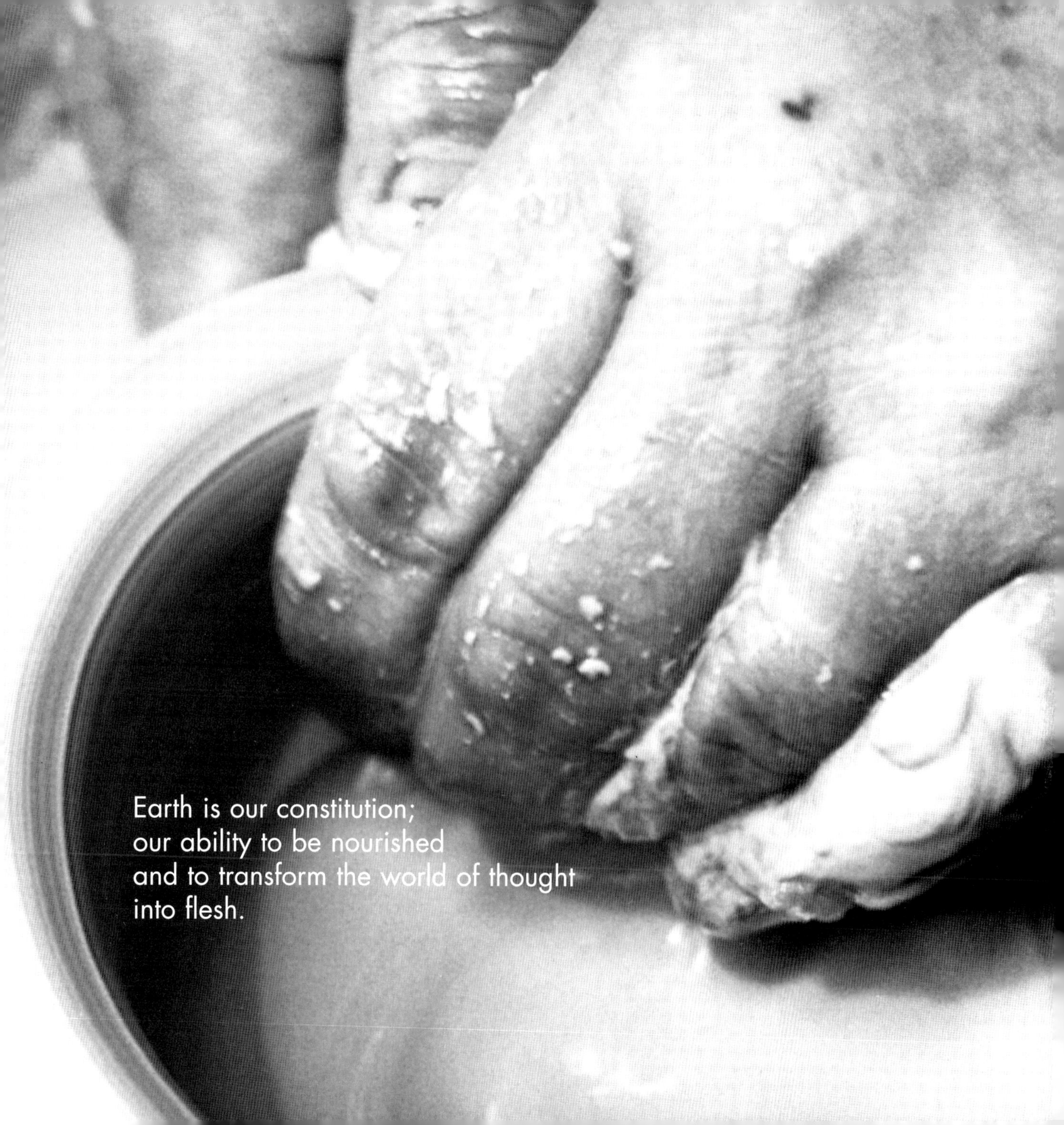
Earth is our constitution;
our ability to be nourished
and to transform the world of thought
into flesh.

Sacred Earth

The energy of the Earth element is acknowledged in our sacred practices through reverence to soil and its qualities. People revere soil not only as a provider but also as a foundation of creation: the Earth element bestows the substances that create our physical form, and in Traditional Chinese Medicine the Earth element governs the flesh — the foundation of the body.

Many of the world's religions, theologies and mythologies speak symbolically of humankind being created from the clay of the Earth — from the very body of the great mother.

Allah made humans from clay, the first being Adam (Koran 32:7, 15:26). Allah sent angels to gather earth which was mixed with fluid to make the clay.

Christians often throw a handful of dirt onto the coffin as a body is committed to the ground. The body is symbolically returned to the element from where it came: the body returns to ashes and dust, the soul to God. In Romans 9:21, God is referred to as the potter with power over the clay that symbolises humans.

Aruru, a goddess in the Babylonian Gilgamesh epic, moulds humans as though they were pots and she the cosmic potter.

Khnum, the ancient Egyptian 'potter god' who created the world, gathers silt from the Nile and makes humans on his great potter's wheel.

Gaia, the Greek Earth Goddess (Mother Nature), existed even before time (one of her many children). She gave humans life from her own fertile womb — from the Earth — and nurtures us with her abundant gifts. She herself was born of Chaos, the great gaping void.

Many voices

The Earth element bestows us with song. In Traditional Chinese Medicine the presence of the sound of song in a person's speaking voice is associated with the presence of Earth element energy.

Our voice can be a tool of nurture and be used to heal; words carry the power of our inner being into the world and share our understanding of life. Songs touch us particularly deeply and a person with strong Earth energy may be given to singing about their innermost feelings or may soothe the hearts of others with a lullaby or song.

Traditionally in many cultures the elders share their knowledge of the spirit of nature and of the ancestors through song. Many indigenous Australians, for instance, understand that the world was sung into being by the ancestors. Song is seen as a creative force in the building of form; people navigate by, and travel on, the songlines of the Earth. These songlines have been likened to the 'energy channels' or 'meridians' of the Earth itself, but in finding common language we don't necessarily find the same understanding. The custodians of the songs teach the spiritual and vocal tradition of songlines to the rightful heirs of the knowledge: the people who belong to that part of the land, who are a part of the land itself.

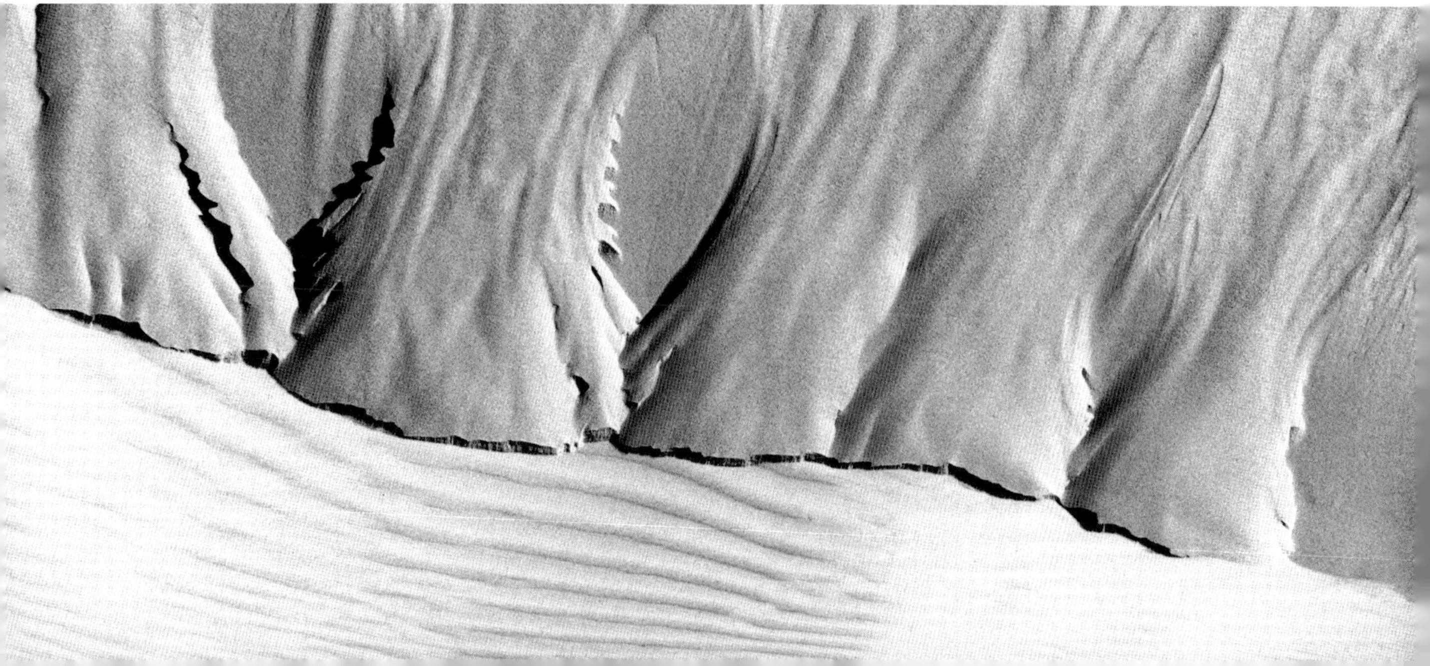

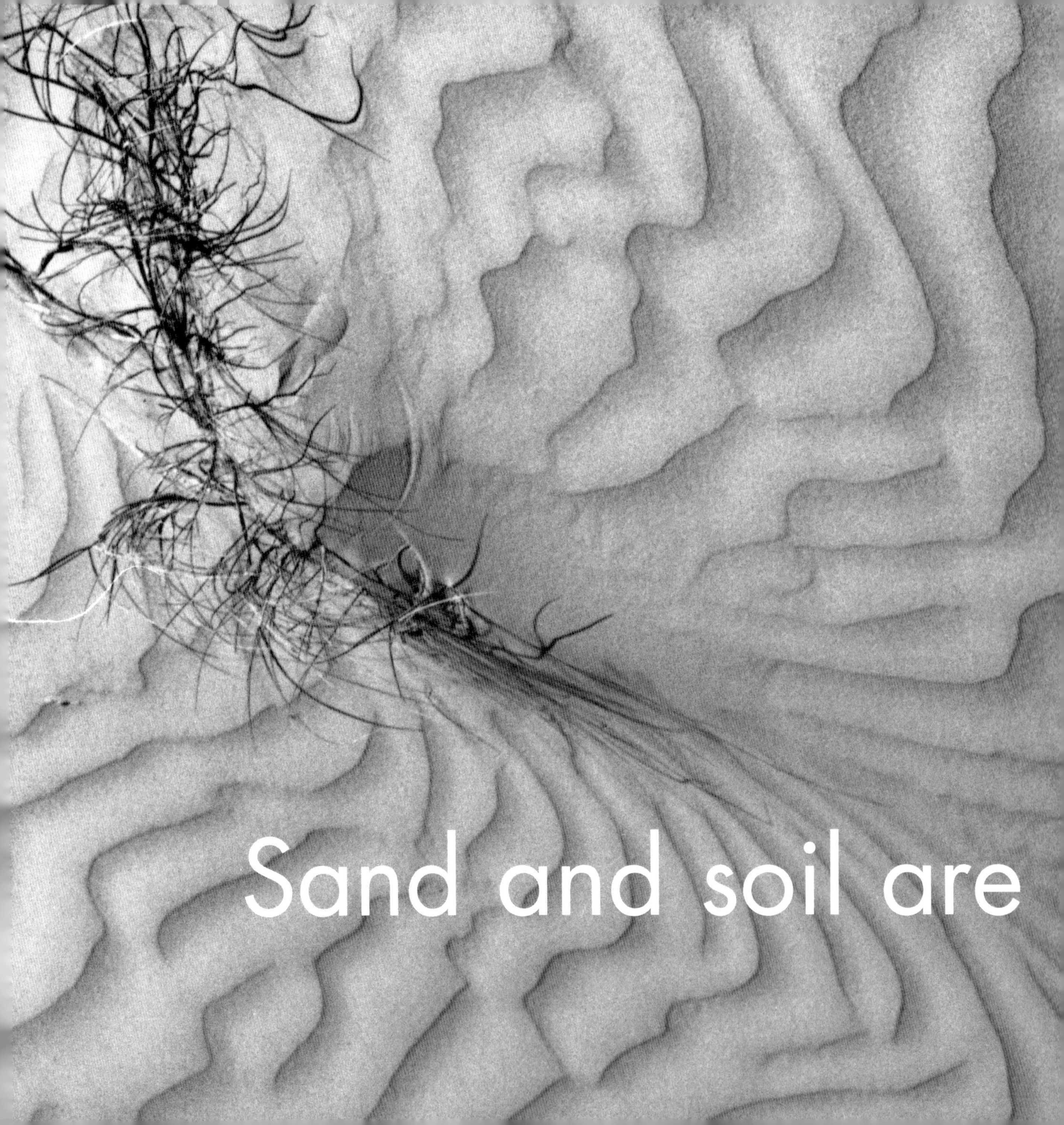

Sand and soil are

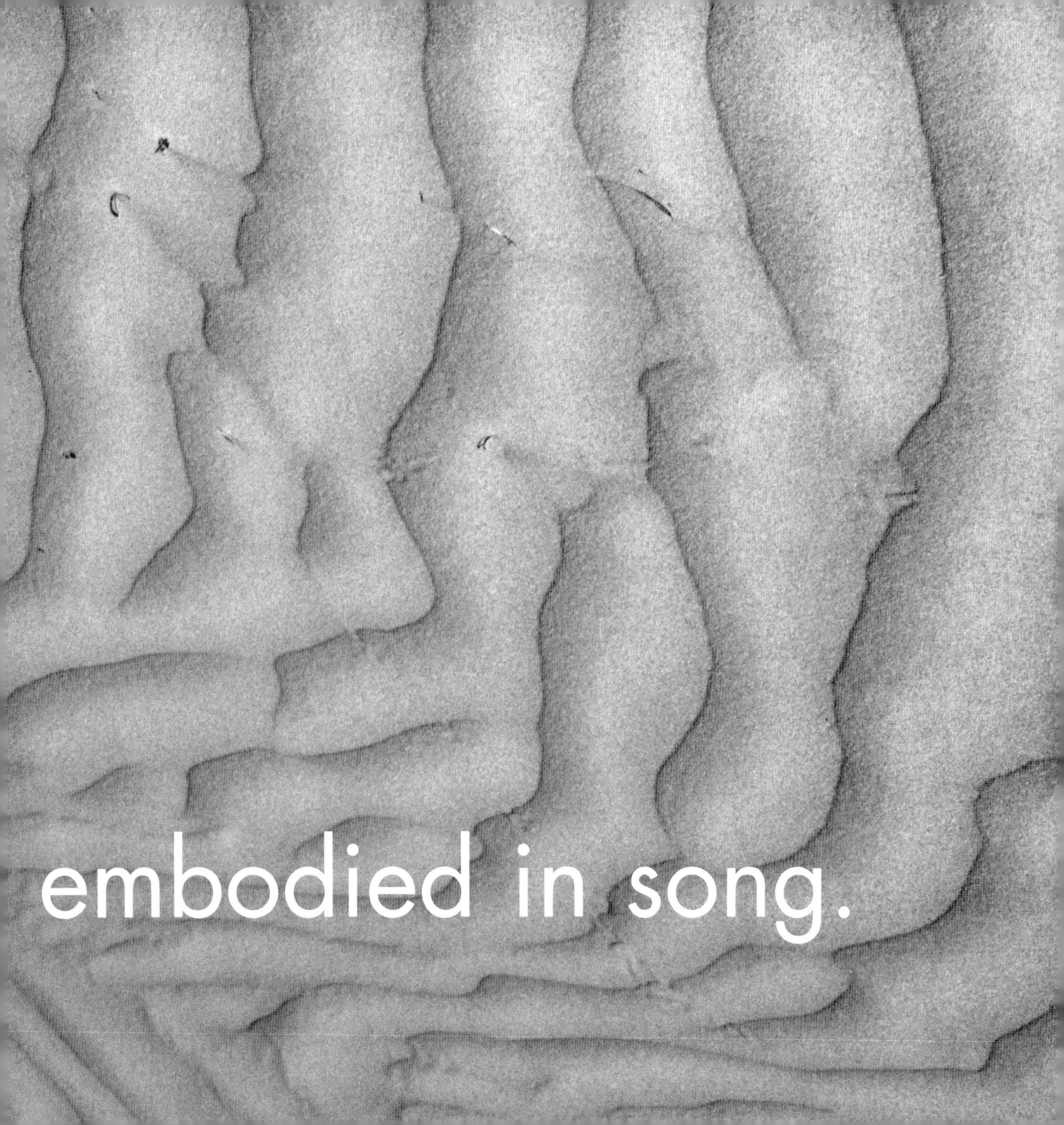
embodied in song.

Compassion

The energy of the Earth element allows the emotion of sympathy and acts of compassion. Both the ability to be compassionate and to receive the compassion of others is traditionally associated with the Earth phase, and extremes involving a lack of compassion, excessive sympathy or neediness are signs of an Earth element imbalance within our bodies.

To feel sorrow for the suffering of others we first need to feel a sense of connection with others. The Earth element reminds us of our shared experience — our shared central point of reference in the vastness of space — and that all of our tears fall on the same planet.

The planet Earth is compassion embodied. Imagine a benign entity with outstretched arms full of material gifts and food. Imagine this entity gathering you up, giving you somewhere safe to lay, and providing the medicines you need and the comfort of touch. This is the nature of the Earth element.

The fuel of compassion

A major function of the Earth element in our bodies is the transformation of what we eat into Qi. The desire to assimilate and transform the world around us in order to nourish our own life force is uncomfortable for some people and they can lose the ability to self-nurture, to 'take in the world'. When we lack the ability to self-nurture we may need great strength from others to overcome feelings of low self-worth and we may find it difficult to nurture in return. In a sense, food is the fuel of compassion, and compassion begins with the act of receiving.

Therapists and caregivers especially need to take time to nurture themselves, to eat good food, and to have some quiet time for meals.

At our foundation is a place of exchange,
where giving and receiving exist as one.

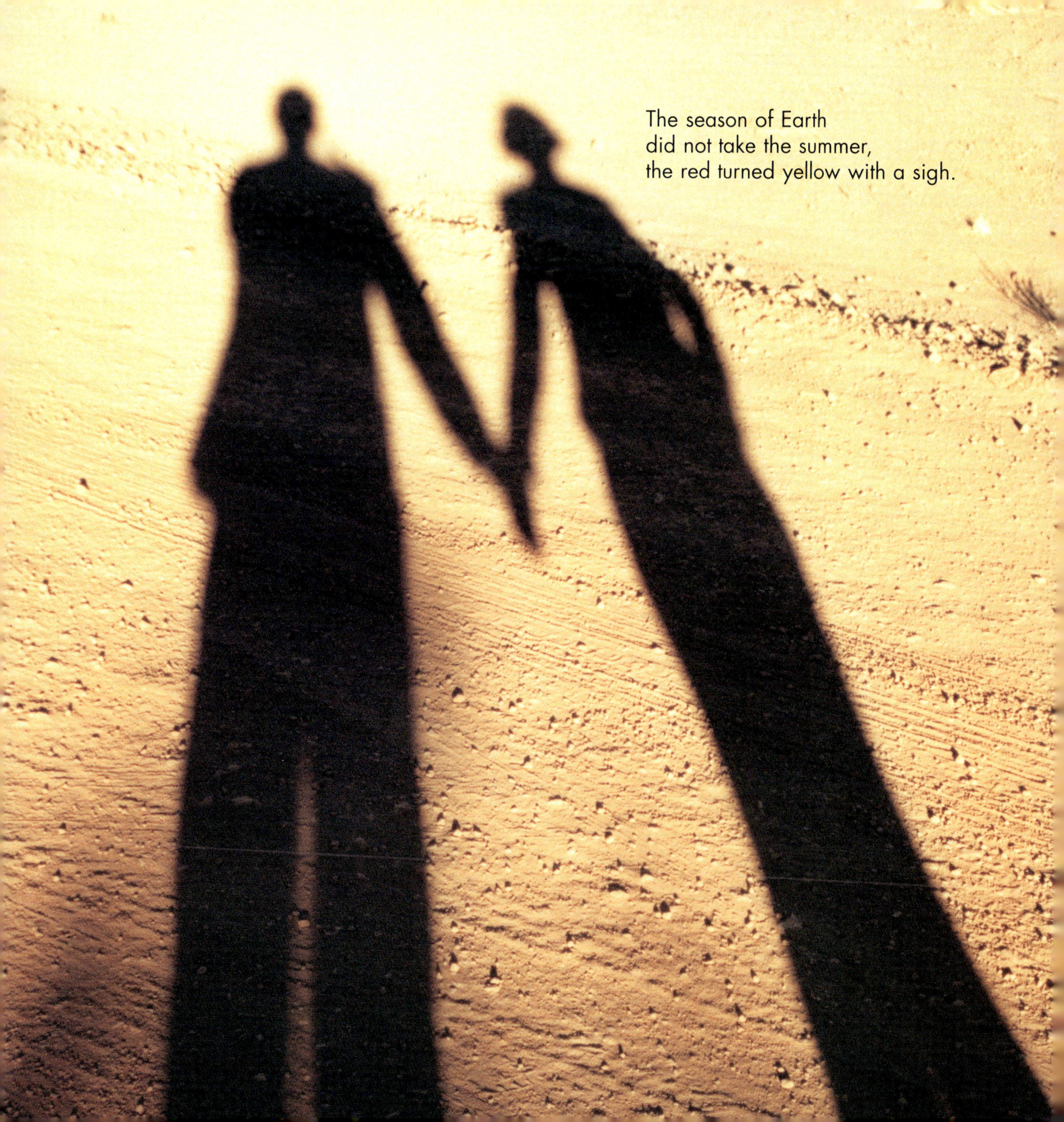

The season of Earth
did not take the summer,
the red turned yellow with a sigh.

In the celestial body of our planet
is the will that creates ascendance.
We, the progeny, are the parents.

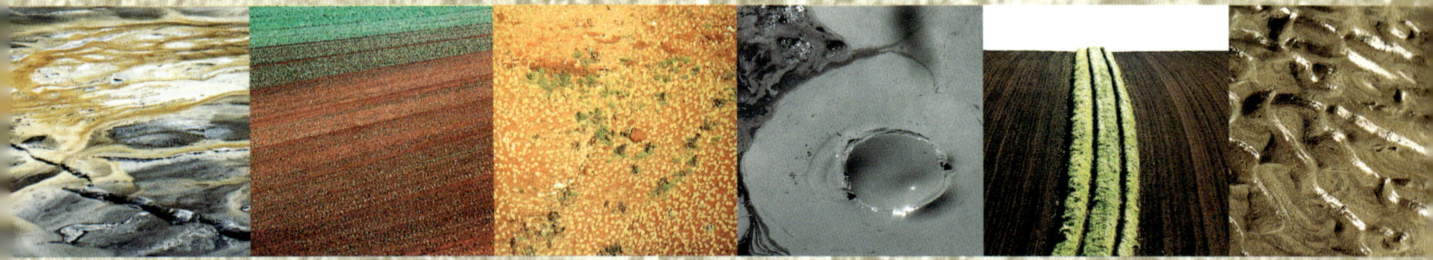

Late summer

The season traditionally associated with the Earth element is late summer. For a moment in the cycle of seasons we pause. Balanced perfectly between the heat of summer and the coming of autumn is a season of solidity, self-realisation and sated calm; the fields have been harvested and the food is safely stored away.

Naturally, seasonal conditions vary according to where we are. In traditional Five Element theory, the Earth element is associated with high humidity in a warm atmosphere. In these conditions vegetable matter begins to mould and rot; the fruits of the earth begin to become overripe and to transform back into earth again. Red, the colour of the Fire element's summer, loses brightness and is replaced with more gentle ochre hues: yellows, browns and shades of orange.

The light softens. Colours merge sympathetically like a water-painted haze. The sun grows smaller as the planet spins on its axis; the afternoon is cooler, temperate and damp. There is time for gratitude and for sharing the fruits of our labours. There is a feeling of coming home to rest and taking stock of our provisions.

Mother and child

The mother element to Earth on the Sheng construction cycle is Fire: Fire is the creator of Earth. Earth in turn is the mother of Metal, but is the representation of the mother as a general concept and as the iconic nurturer.

In the control or destruction cycle of the Five Element theory, the Earth element is the control of Water and offers a metaphor for the effects of being overly protective or overcontrolling: the Earth smothers the Water, entraps it and stagnates it. This can be visualised with images of a muddy puddle, a silted river or a dam that has nothing to feed it.

When the Earth energy within us is healthy we give freely of ourselves. In Traditional Chinese Medicine the stomach channel is associated with the Earth element and runs right down the front of our body through each breast. One of the points on this channel is located in each nipple. Earth is literally and metaphorically the source of nourishment and bestows us with the milk of life.

Meditation on Earth

Let your body and mind come to rest in this moment and place, sitting comfortably in your meditation posture. Have your eyes softly open, focused on the ground just ahead of you. Your lips are lightly closed, and the tip of your tongue rests against the top palate of your mouth.

Place your hands, fingertips touching, either side of your navel. You can use a pillow on your lap or a 'meditation belt' made from a meditation shawl with the knot to the front to support your hands.

Bring your attention to your breathing. Watch your breath as it moves in and out of your body, and feel the expansion of your belly. Feel the breath push your fingertips apart.

Let the in-breath inspire a feeling of fulfilment in your belly. The in-breath will naturally part your fingertips as your belly expands.

As you breathe out, feel your body surrender to gravity. Surrender completely without collapsing; you are relaxed, yet you are upright.

The sound on your out-breath is like a sighing note of a song and carries a feeling of letting go. Just let go.

Your fingertips will naturally touch again at the end of the out-breath, and the area around your navel may feel like it has 'butterflies', as when you're in love.

Stay with these images for a time until your breathing is easy and full.

Release all your tension on the sighing out-breath. Let go. This is an immensely safe place.

Shift your attention now and choose a person in your life to send a thought of loving-kindness to, perhaps a friend or family member. You may choose a person you have difficulty with, or someone in need of nurture and healing.

Bring this person's name to mind on the in-breath, and send them loving thoughts on the out: 'be well and happy'. Try not to become involved in thoughts about your relationship with this person. Just send love.

When your meditation nears an end, return to watching your breath as it moves in and out of your body. Gradually slow the movement of your breath until it is so gentle it is almost imperceptible. Feel the fullness in your belly.

Lay down quietly before rising and perhaps allow yourself to fall asleep.

During the day contemplate the qualities of compassion and kindness.

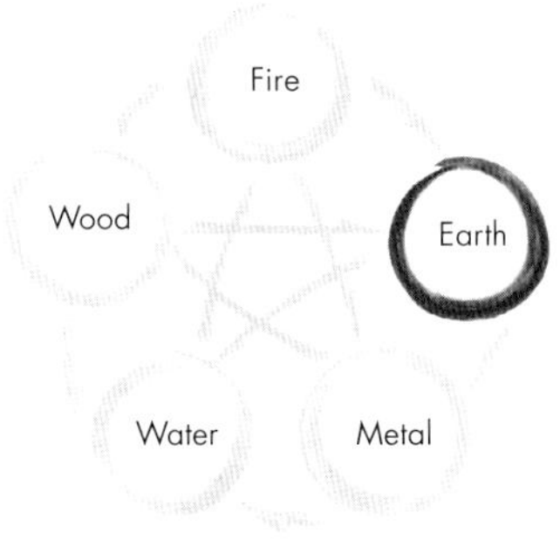

Earth energy in Traditional Chinese Medicine

The Minister of Food

I am the Minister of Food, transforming the materials needed to nourish all the elements. I am abundant; my destiny is to provide for the physical and emotional needs of myself and others. I am at the middle of and central to the production of the body's energy. I am the Earth element.

The Earth element channels and important points

The Earth element has two channels of Qi flow in the body. These channels are named after the organs most directly associated with the Earth element: *stomach* and *spleen*. The *stomach* channel begins just under the eye and travels down the face and throat, through the abdomen and down the outside of the leg, finishing at the nail of the second toe. The *spleen* channel starts at the outside of the big toe and traverses up the inside of the leg, penetrates the abdomen and finishes in the chest.

- *Zusanli*, meaning 'Three Leg Distance', brings me energy as it is the main point to strengthen the *stomach* and *spleen* organs and Qi. This point helps digestion and builds strength and immunity. It is perhaps the most commonly used point when there is any type of weakness in the body and is the thirty-sixth point on the stomach channel.

- If my weakness is of the blood and I have menstrual problems or pain in my abdomen, then *Sanyinjiao* is a point that can benefit. Translated as 'Three Yin Intersection', it is the sixth point on the *spleen* channel and is where the *kidney*, *liver* and *spleen* channels cross over. I can call on the healing attributes of all three channels with this one point.
- *Baihui*, translated as 'Hundred Meetings', is at the top of the head and it is where many channels converge. When I feel heavy and tired and can't think straight it can help raise my energy and clear my mind. This point also lessens the effects of gravity on my body by raising the Qi that holds things in place.

Earth element channels in the body

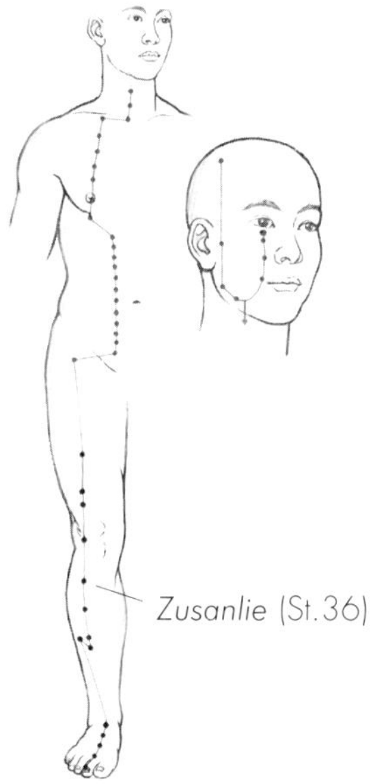

Stomach — Yang channel of Earth

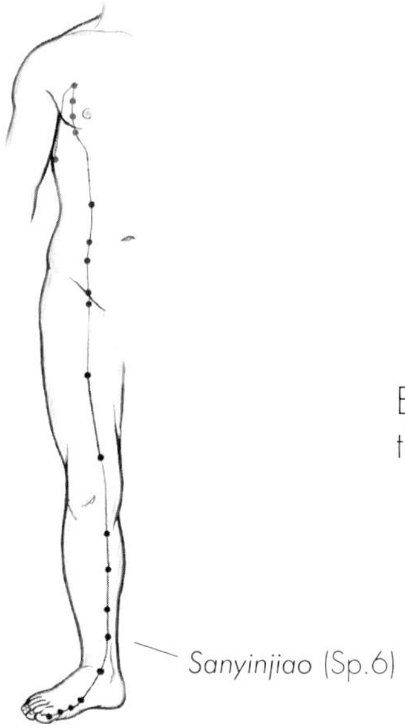

Spleen — Yin channel of Earth

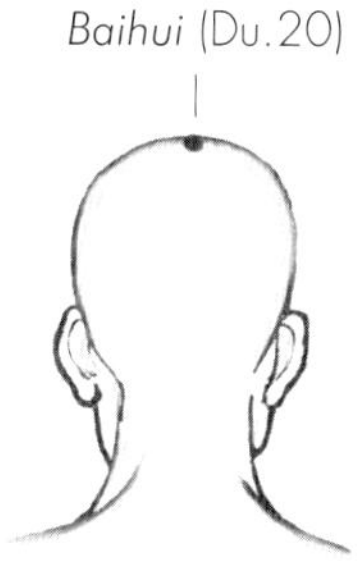

Extra point on the Du channel

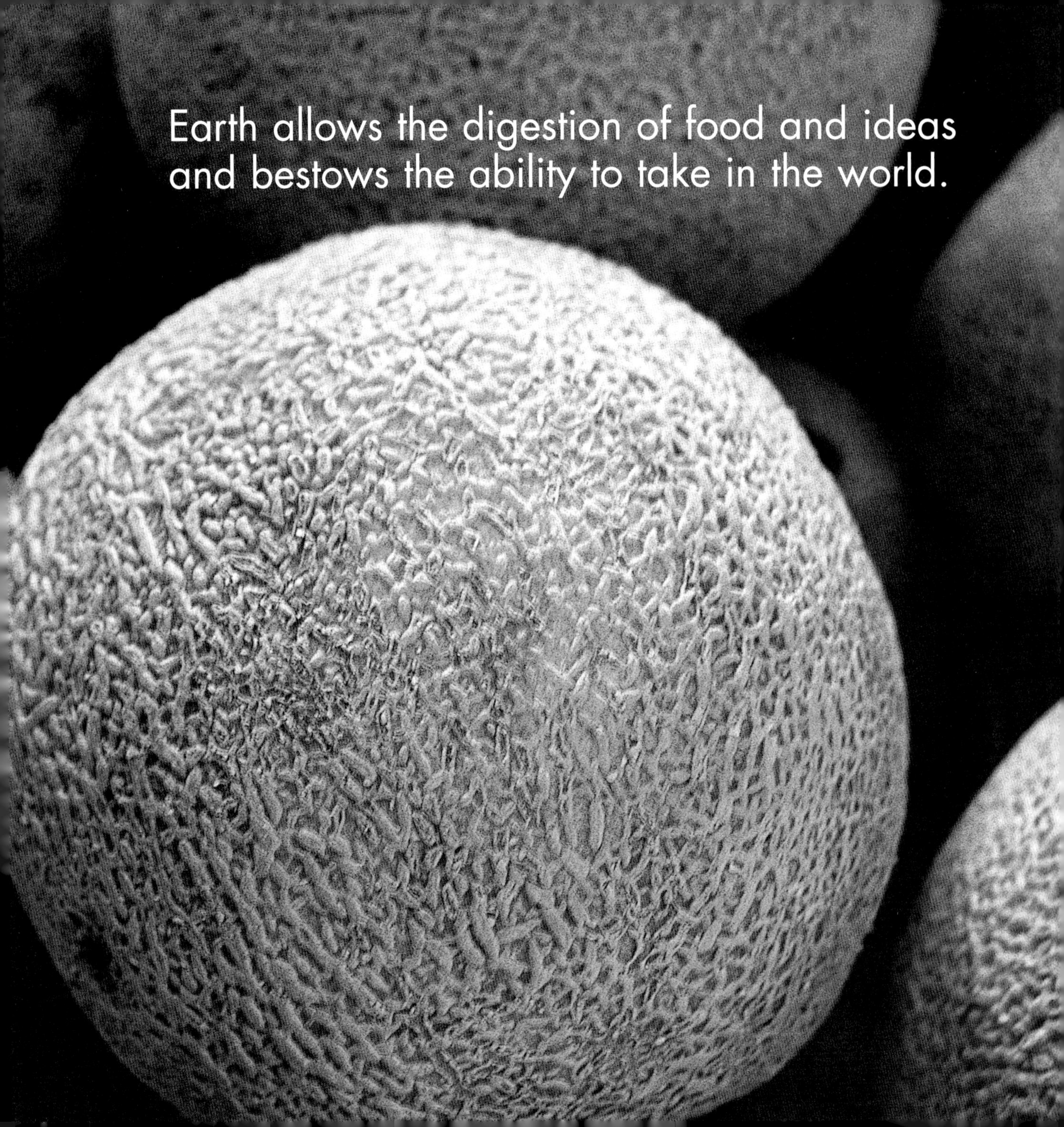

Earth allows the digestion of food and ideas and bestows the ability to take in the world.

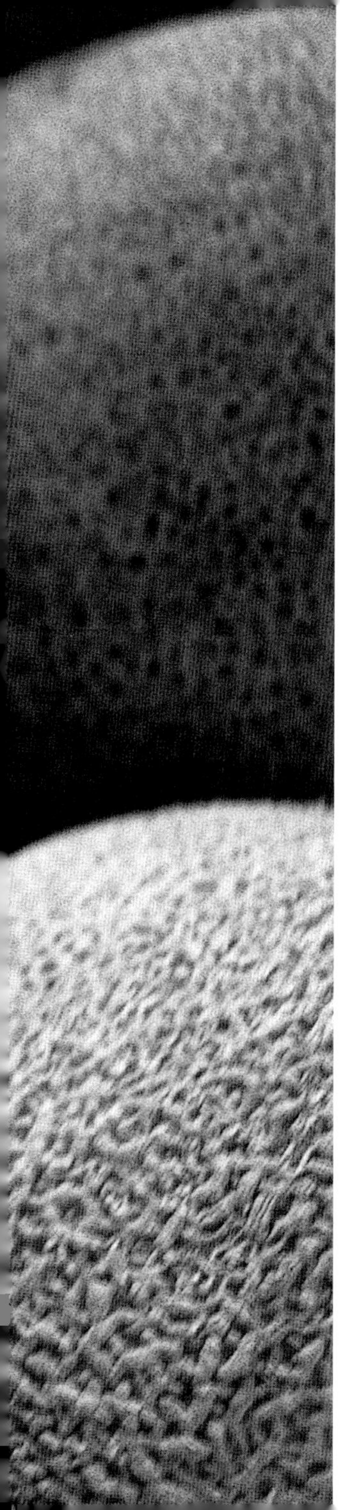

The Earth element within our body, mind and emotions

Body

The stomach and the spleen are the coupled organs of my Earth element and have many attributed functions in Traditional Chinese Medicine that transcend the ideas of an organ's basic mechanical function. The direction of Qi movement in the *stomach* and *spleen* channels is opposite to one another. *Stomach* Qi naturally moves downwards and *spleen* Qi moves upwards. This forms a central field that counteracts the forces of gravity in my body. When I feel 'heavy' and am drawn to lie down it can mean my *spleen* Qi is no longer pushing upwards. Nausea is a sign that my *stomach* Qi is going upwards when it really wants to go downwards. When all is in balance the *spleen* energy transforms the distilled essence of my stomach's hard work to give me a special type of nourishing Qi.

In Traditional Chinese Medicine, Earth governs my sense of taste and produces the blood. Dark spots in my vision can mean a weakness in the blood, as can low self-esteem. In strengthening the blood, self-esteem issues are benefited along with other Earth attributes.

My Earth element is responsible for keeping all the other organs in their rightful positions and my blood within my vessels. Earth also governs flesh and the shape of my body. Low appetite means there is not enough *spleen* channel energy to digest my food whereas Fire in the stomach creates hunger.

Mind

Contemplation is a key virtue of my Earth element, but worry or excessive thinking will deplete me, causing a scattering of my energies. If I lose my centre I can become obsessed by real or imagined scarcity. As a fast learner, mindfulness and concentration are my strengths and I digest ideas easily. Being fixated is a sign that my Earth is not processing ideas, and poor concentration signals that my Earth's resources are low.

Emotions

Sympathy and caring are attributes of my Earth element. These qualities form the central core around which the other emotions gather. Those in need sense my genuine concern for their lack. As I patiently listen and give generously of my time I can easily lose sight of my own emotional needs or even lose sight of whose problem belongs to whom. I myself can succumb to needy behaviour when my Earth energy is depleted. If I am unable to digest ideas properly I will go over my problems in a circular manner with those who have enough Earth energy to listen — but be aware that I don't seek a solution, I seek sympathy. The lesson here is that sometimes it is better to throw a lifeline to someone who has fallen overboard than to jump in with them. At this point sympathy becomes compassion and real help can be given.

Destiny of the Earth element

My destiny is to bring abundance to the other elements in order to complete them. I balance the elements through contemplation and fulfil their needs where I sense lack. I assimilate ideas easily and through mindfulness I transform sympathy into the more highly refined virtue of compassion, thereby completing myself.

Thought and fire
take body in the soil.
Earth is intent on form.

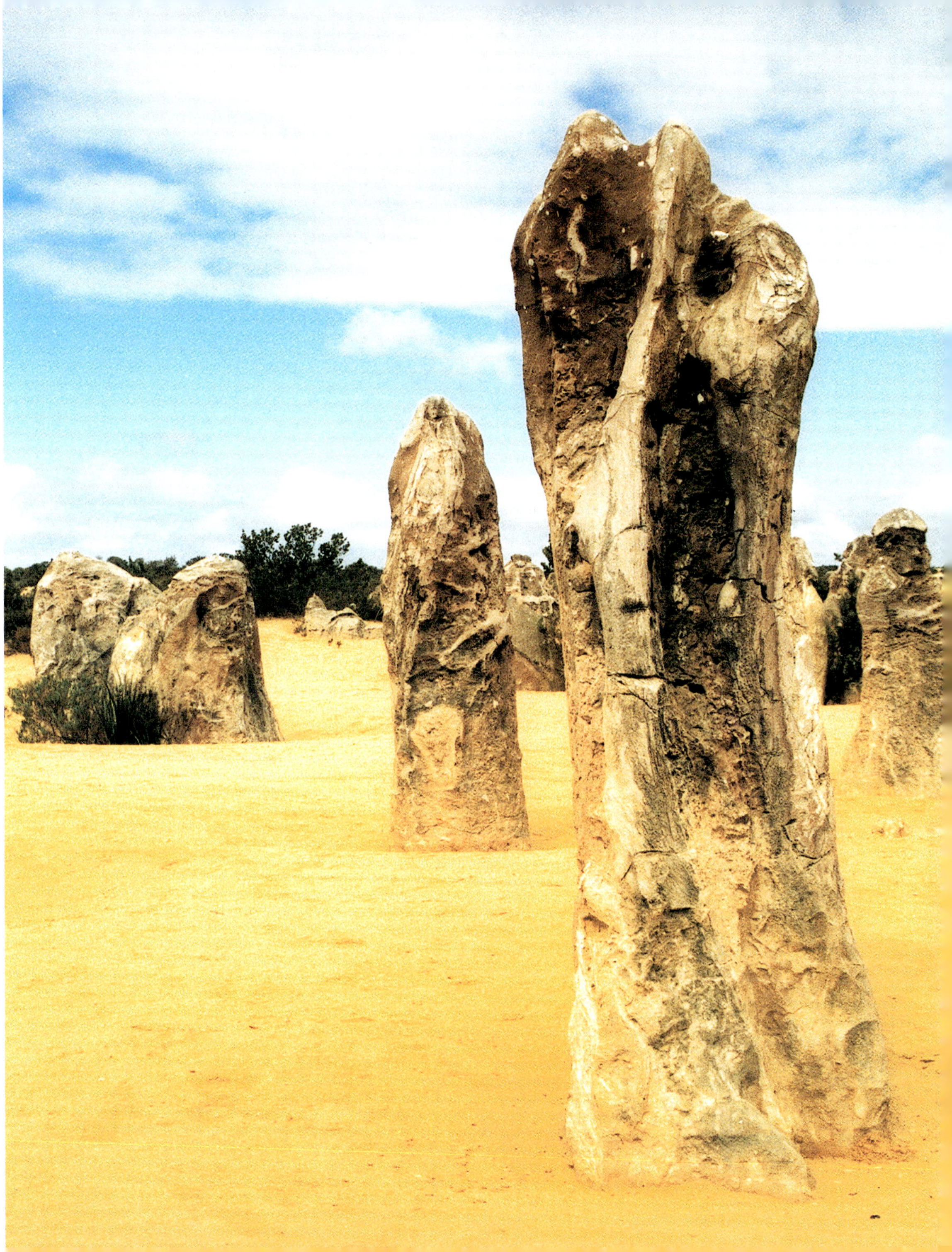

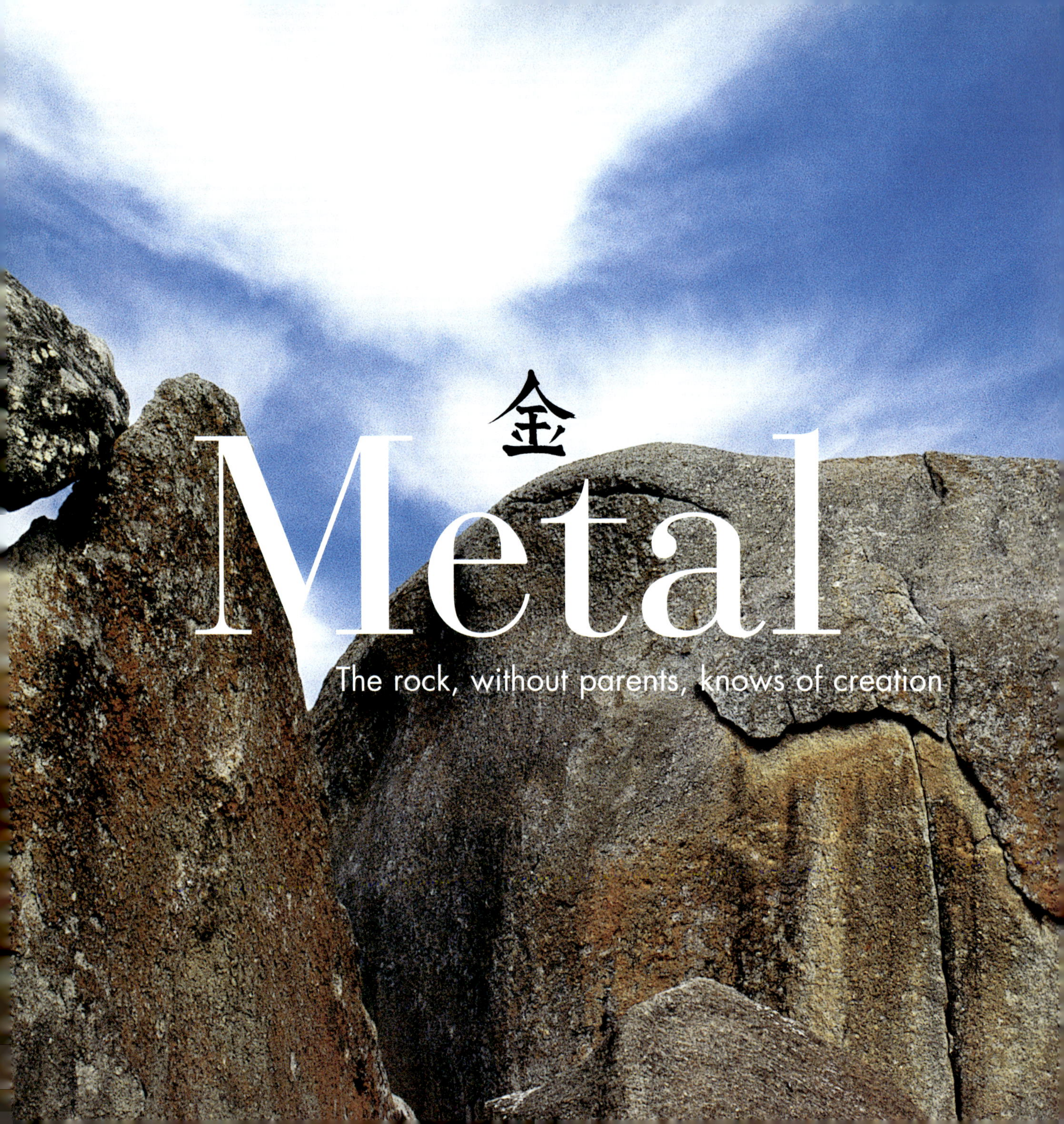

金

Metal

The rock, without parents, knows of creation

Metal

In all maturity is this, my objective awareness.
I am the ultimate manifestation of matter,
the sacred place revered by all,
the inorganic form.
Unmoved.
I am the centre of self-knowledge without judgement.
I measure time from this first breath to this last.
I stand aside and free the same self
from my surroundings;
not withdrawing.
I understand the beauty of numbers and absolutes,
yet am transcendental in my learning,
with no concern for passion.
I am melancholic
and wise.
I am the subject of human spiritual pilgrimage
and the backbone of all economy.
My sibling's name is gravity;
we understand weight
and density.
I am now and forever the quintessential point,
existing in the cosmic breath.
I have no lineage.
No parent.
No seed.
I do not understand subjection or sympathy.
My silver moon mirrors and reflects;
the soul world is a reality.
I am Metal.

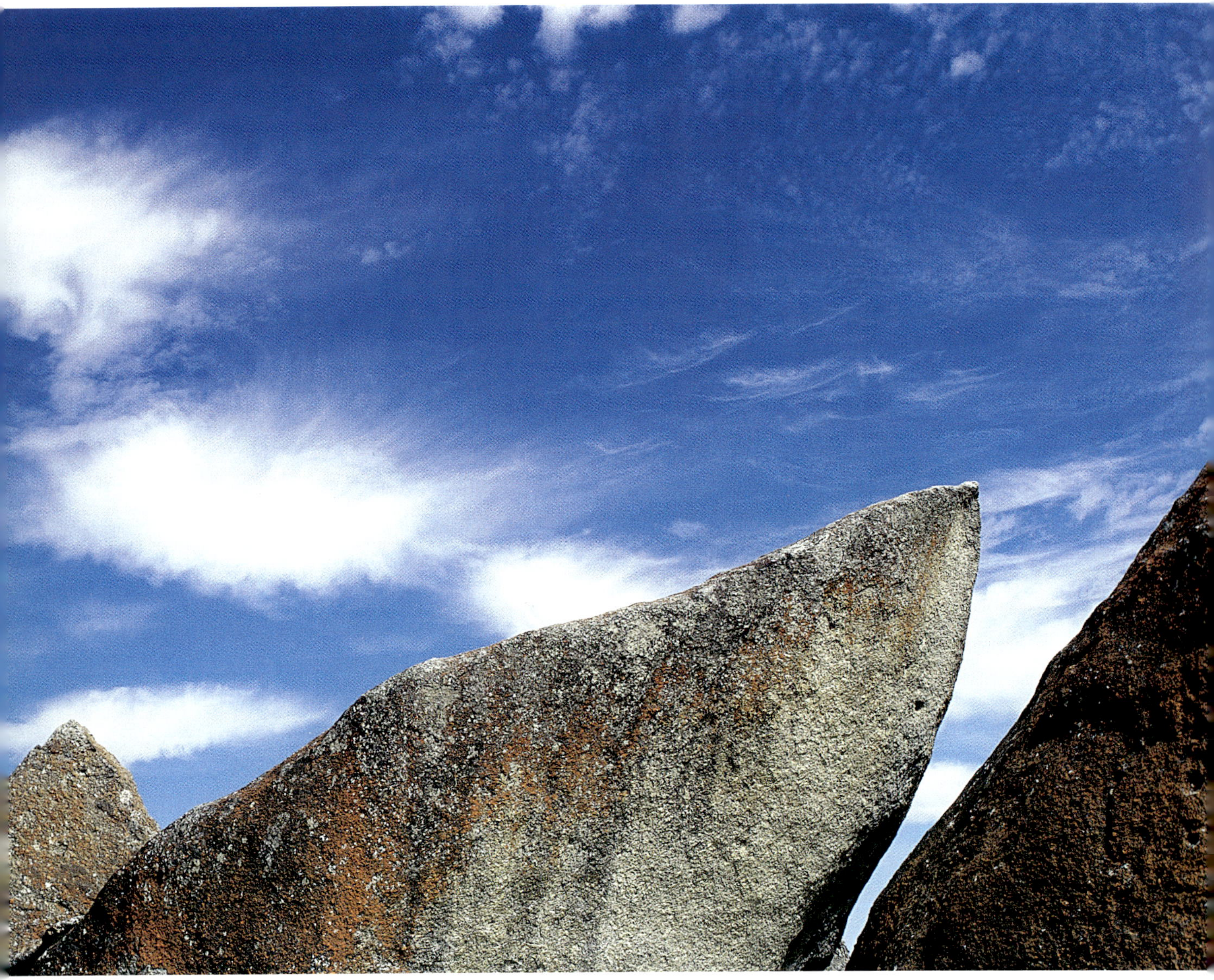

Traditional Chinese Metal element associations:

Autumn, white, weeping and grief, hair and skin, the nose, dryness, the lungs, the large intestine, the pungent flavours, the direction of west.

The Metal element expressed in nature

In nature the Metal phase of creation takes form in mountains, rocks, stones and ores. These substances represent the qualities of Metal well: Metal is fundamental, primary, inscrutable, and consolidated.

The Metal element draws mass and matter into dynamically compressed points of reference and creates definite boundaries. Metal may seem detached and complete unto itself. It can stand alone like a rock in the ocean that looks objectively at the moving world around it. The mountain rising up from the plains is an awe-inspiring display of independence as it watches over the lands below from lofty heights. But Metal is not inert or autonomous; it actively interacts with the world.

Metal is the mother of Water in the creation cycle. Metal 'holds' and supports water and allows water to be embodied in a system of interconnected streams, rivers and oceans. Water flows in the canyons and stone riverbeds, chattering and burbling as it passes between the rocks, conducted on its way by the power of Metal.

Orbiting the earth (the mother of Metal in the Wu Xing), the moon watches over its own prodigy, Water, and creates the rise and fall of tides — the lifting and releasing of oceans. Seemingly lifeless and in itself still, the moon silently communes with the waters and the earth, knowing the secrets of space.

The moon is a natural (but not traditional) symbol for the power of the Metal element. This ancient battered ball of rock does not rotate to show the secret side; it symbolically presents an unchanging face that reflects upon the earth, offering the constant assuredness of something other. When we look to this face we feel a connection with the realms beyond our daylight world and a melancholic draw to the coolness of silent communication. The moon is like a cosmic mirror that reflects the ways of the world. It is the physical symbol for 'that which is outside ourself' — the silent friend who shows us ourselves with an objective clarity.

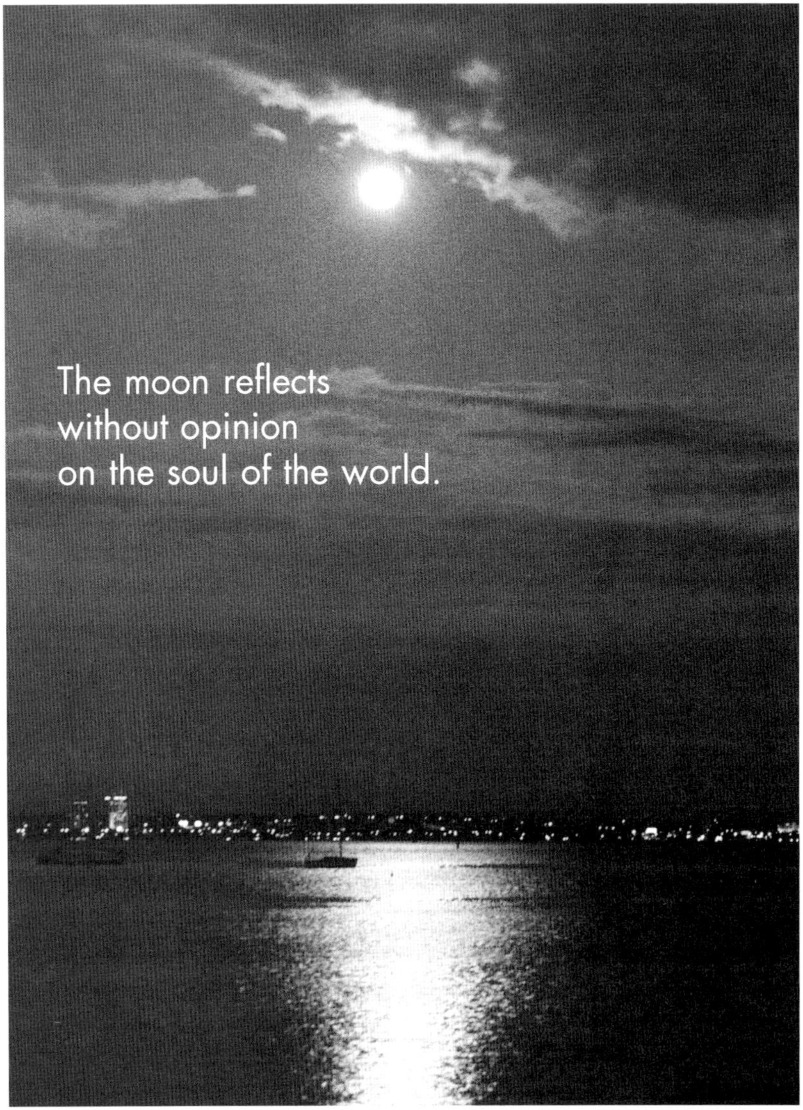
The moon reflects
without opinion
on the soul of the world.

In Five Element theory, Metal breathes the air of heaven and brings inspiration to the world. Metal is imbued with the knowledge of places beyond this planet; it is a symbol of a space where a continuous 'in-breath' and 'out-breath' meet in a moment of perfect stillness and harmony. Metal creates the idea of timeless immediacy and allows the flow of pure 'air Qi' in our bodies.

Inspiration and expiration

The last organs to develop in a foetus are the lungs — the Yin organ associated with the Metal element. Unlike other organs, the lungs don't begin to truly function until they are exposed to the atmosphere. As we inhale and exhale we gain a primary connection with our world. Through the lungs comes the first sign and measure of our earthly life — our first in-breath — and the designated end of earthly life — our last out-breath.

As we breathe we gather inspiration for life. The lung organs are the softest and most membranous tissue matter that we expose to the outside world; they are intrinsic to the idea of 'taking in the world'. They allow us an exchange — a sacred link — with our environment and are our rawest relationship with it. In particular, we share a symbiotic relationship with vegetation as we exchange oxygen and carbon dioxide and are sensitive to disruptions in the balance of our atmospheric mixture. It takes only seconds for a disruption in our oxygen intake to have serious consequences: clean air is a constant requirement for our health.

When we breathe deeply we activate Qi. This Qi brings rhythm and stability to our being and inspires our body towards health and balance. It also strengthens the body's structure and brings a feeling of reverent peace to our being.

Metal is the channel for communication that does not hold to words alone.

Humankind and Metal

In the industrious aspects of our lives — in the world of communication and manufacture — metal underpins our activities. Interconnection is an important aspect of Metal; we use metals to relay messages and to keep in touch. The metaphysical power of metal lends itself to the design of systems that send images and voices along cables or through thin air. Metal is the material of the sender and the receiver, allowing free congress of information through conduction. Metal is the conductor of the orchestra — of the orchestrated — and is the wisely impartial interpreter of the invisible voice.

The material of the currency we exchange is metal. Gold and silver rank highly in the metal nobility tables, while diamonds and sapphires typify our love of the precious, of things most pure and rare. We enjoy the exquisite nature of objects so seamless and inorganic; we marvel that nature has taken millions of years to perfect each one. Currency is about exchange and is symbolic of Metal's intention to convey. Metal passes currents, and currency, from one place to another.

The occult value of metallic substances is understood in every culture on earth. Stones may heal spiritual or emotional maladies; metals may ensure health through contact as jewellery; ancestors and gods may dwell in the deities of rock; a crystal formation may have, or represent, the power of healing and magic. An alchemist seeks knowledge of metals and the secrets of its transmutation. Alchemy walks a delicious path between science and the occult and freely engages both as inseparable in a quest to understand nature.

Iron provides a crude material for manufacture. Metal by its nature consolidates, offering us a material that is strongly independent of its physical surroundings. Steel holds shape; it can be made into tools and weapons that bring force to bear against the other elements. A sword or axe is revered for its unrelenting nature and ability to exert influence over the organic — particularly wood — through the impartiality of its substance. However, all of the elements have their 'control' and metal turns to liquid in the presence of Fire!

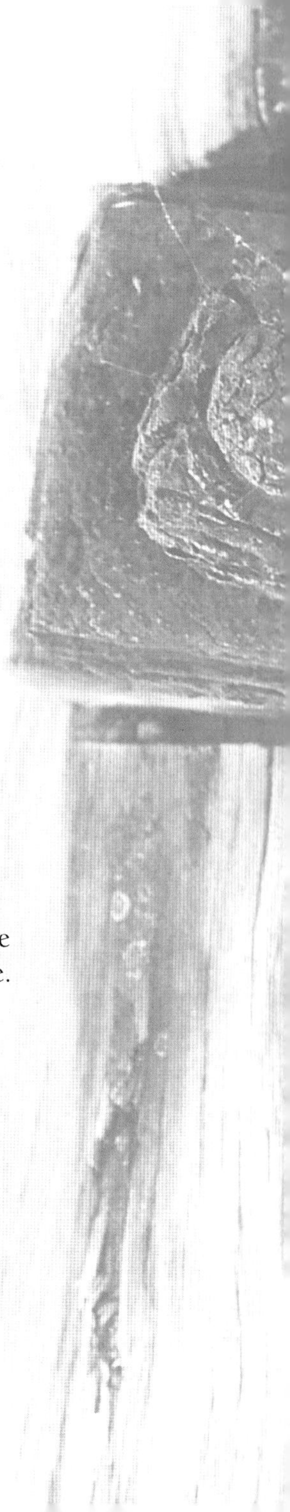

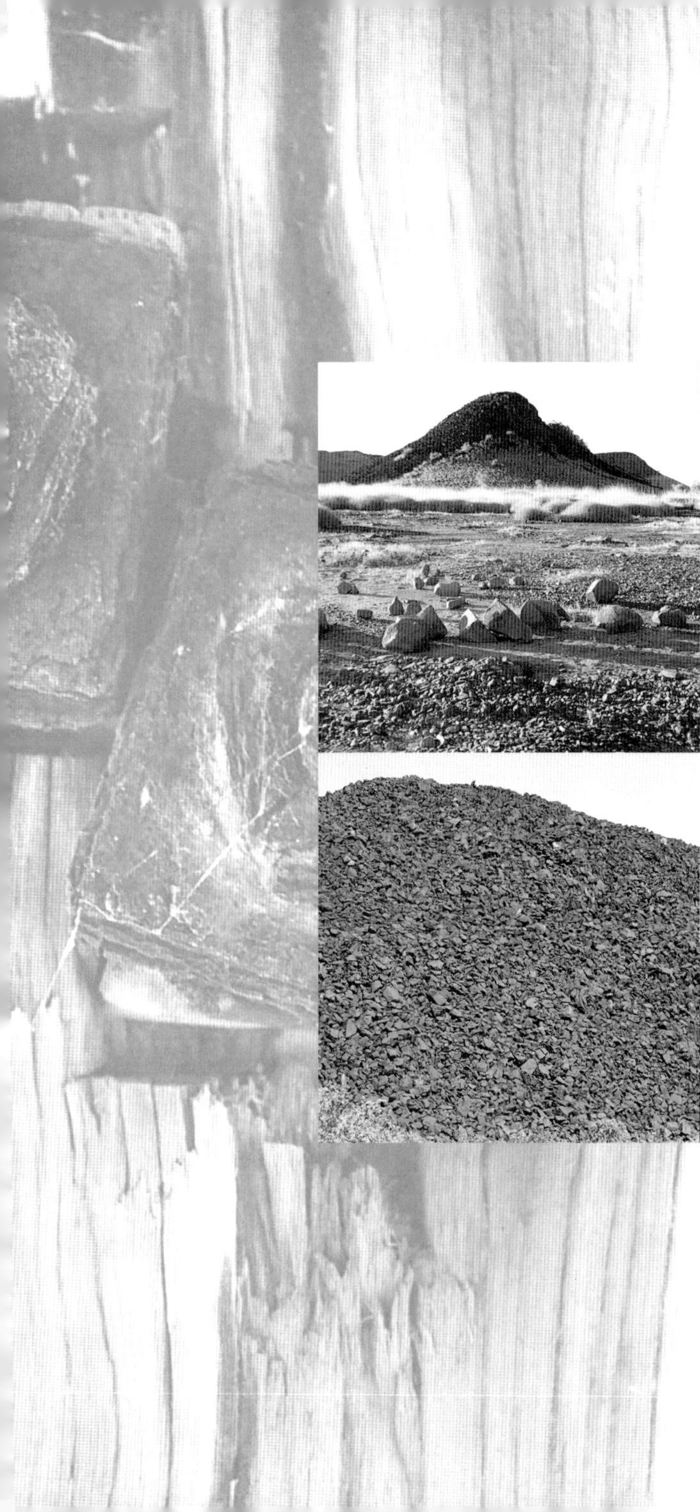

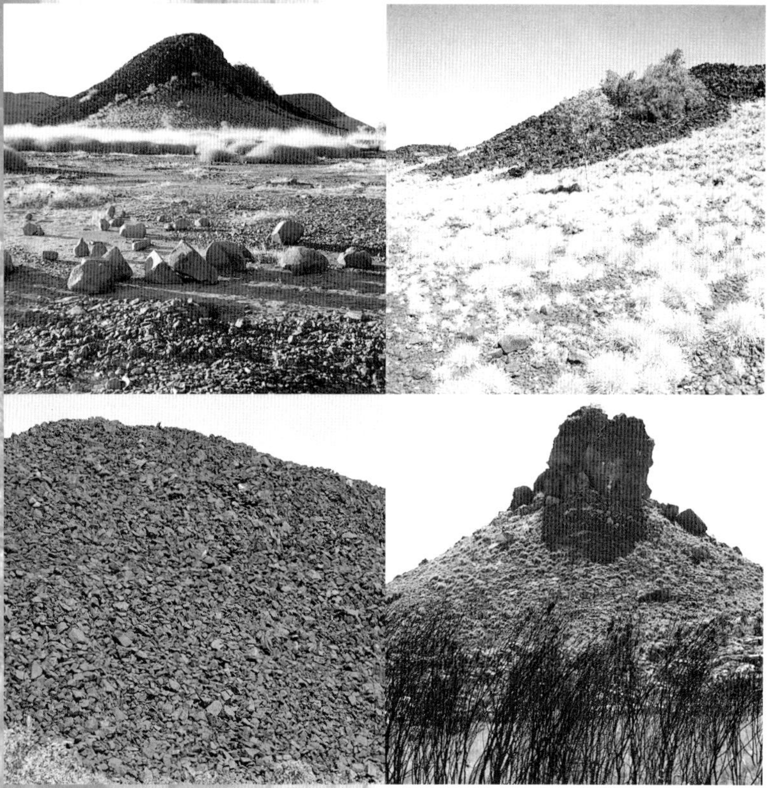

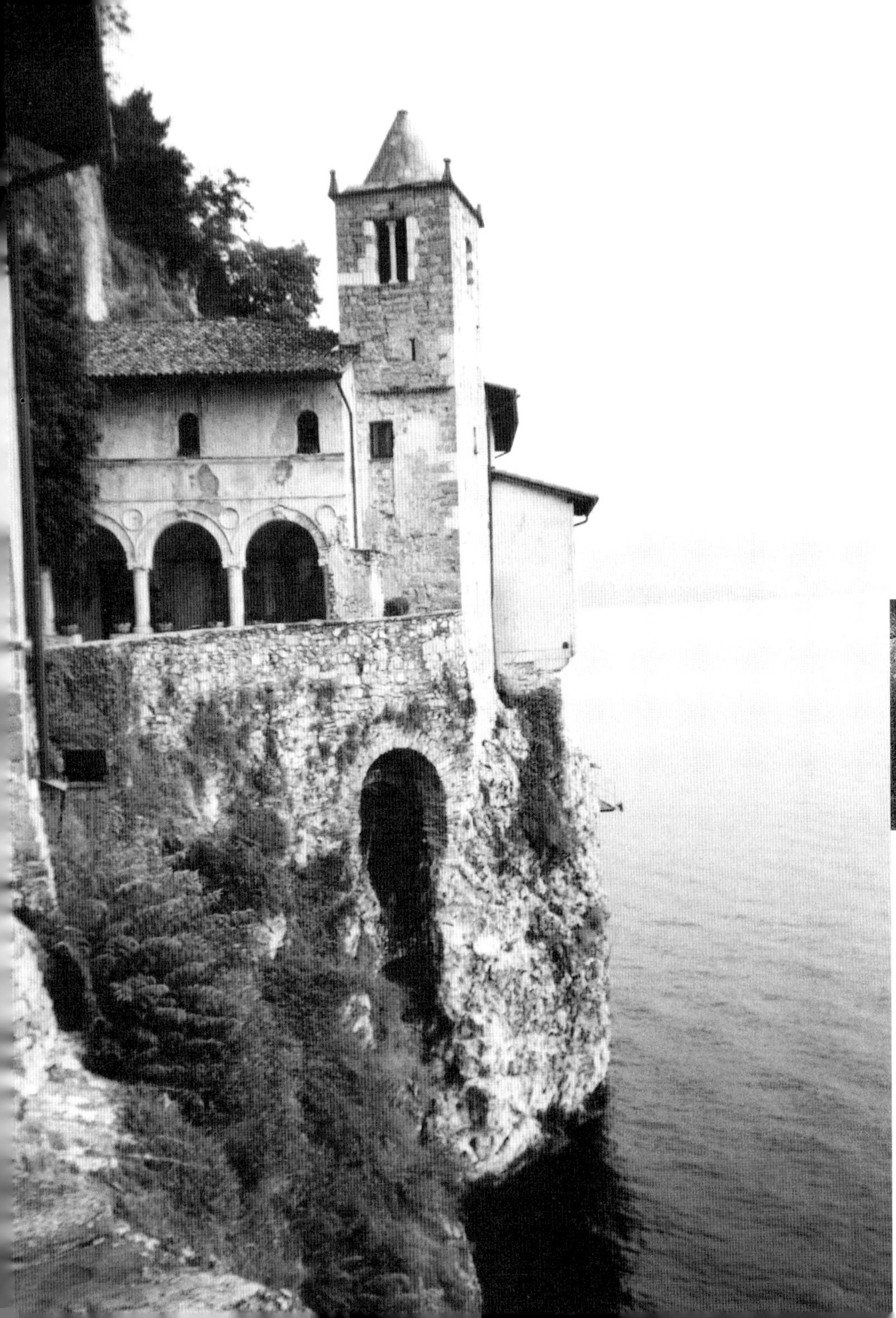

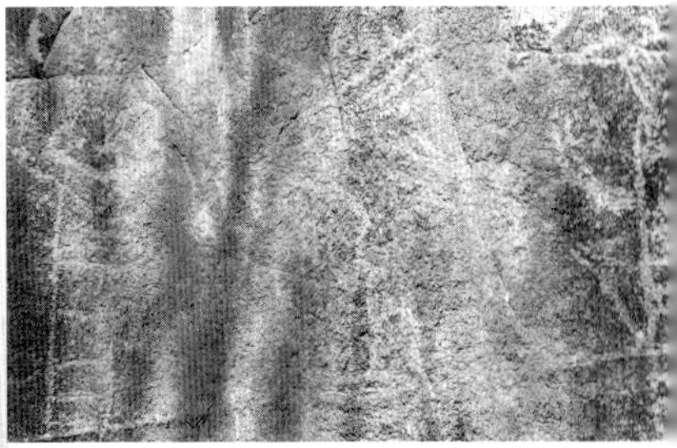

Sacred Metal

The energy of Metal is concerned with the sacred nature and the spiritual aspirations of humans. Our use of stone and metal offers wonderful untraditional symbolism for the spiritual qualities of the Metal element.

The temple high in the mountains is a world of solitude, of wisdom, of transcendence — and of Metal energy. Here we seek to be away from the desires and attractions of joyful Fire, the controller of Metal. In this place the solemnity of life is as focused as the forces within the boulders that make the walls. Here we can travel into an inner world and seek the objective nature of our unnamed being.

The cathedral reminds us of the nature of reverence and the feeling of peace associated with the knowledge that there are great forces at work. We may feel connected with places beyond the visible world and enjoy the solemn nature of silent communication — the meditative power of prayer.

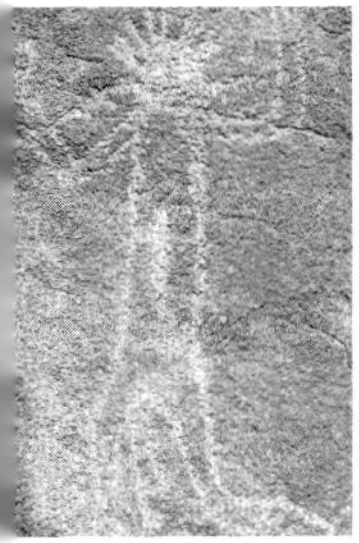

Caves are also places of introspection and departure from the physical world of light and colour into the world of transcendence. People seeking solitude, retreat and meditation may leave behind even the temple to be in a cave.

In many cultures caves are the places where the stories and knowledge of the ancestors are recorded in images. The caves where these paintings and carvings exist are often sacred places concerned with cultural and spiritual teaching and with rites of passage.

The tablet imparts and preserves the messages we received from our meditations and spiritual communications. Tablets are sometimes given the esoteric attributes of actually having been written in the heavens before being passed into the world of humans. The imagery echoes the role Metal plays in our quest for divine communion.

If we value a message we inscribe it in stone. To be written in stone gives a word the strength of preservation, and the weight of being imbued with great merit.

The monument shows human reverence for the dead. Gravestones, tombs and mighty pyramids symbolise the solemnity of the event and the stillness of the eternal. Stone can inspire feelings of permanence and of connection with unearthly life.

Borders

The Metal element governs the act of worldly interaction (interconnection) and the ability to set boundaries at the same time. The nature of transmission and communication is also the nature of separateness — the ability to perceive what is within, and what is without. Skin, under the control of the Metal element, offers a very tactile image for this interaction.

Skin is our first outward contact with the world, but is also our first physical barrier. It distinguishes our body from the world by offering a definitive outer limit to our body. Our skin also offers defence and immunity when the body is healthy, and is constantly exchanging fluid levels with the atmosphere while breathing through the pores.

The delicate act of receiving and rejecting simultaneously is not the juggling of two acts; it is the extraordinary ability of Metal to perform the role of exchange and embodiment as a unified intention.

Metal creates a mysterious point
of consolidated matter,
where a continuous in-breath
and out-breath merge together.

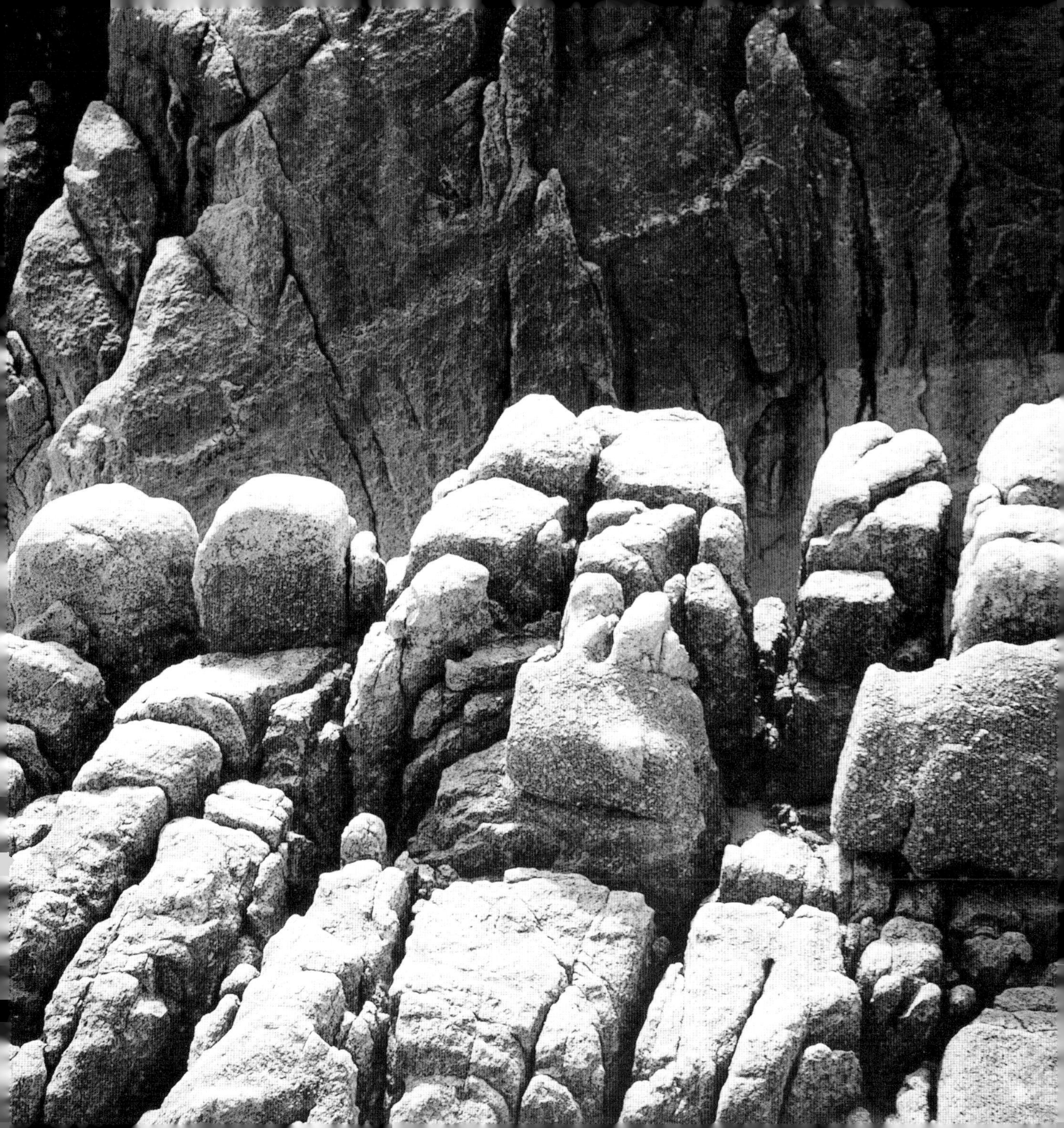

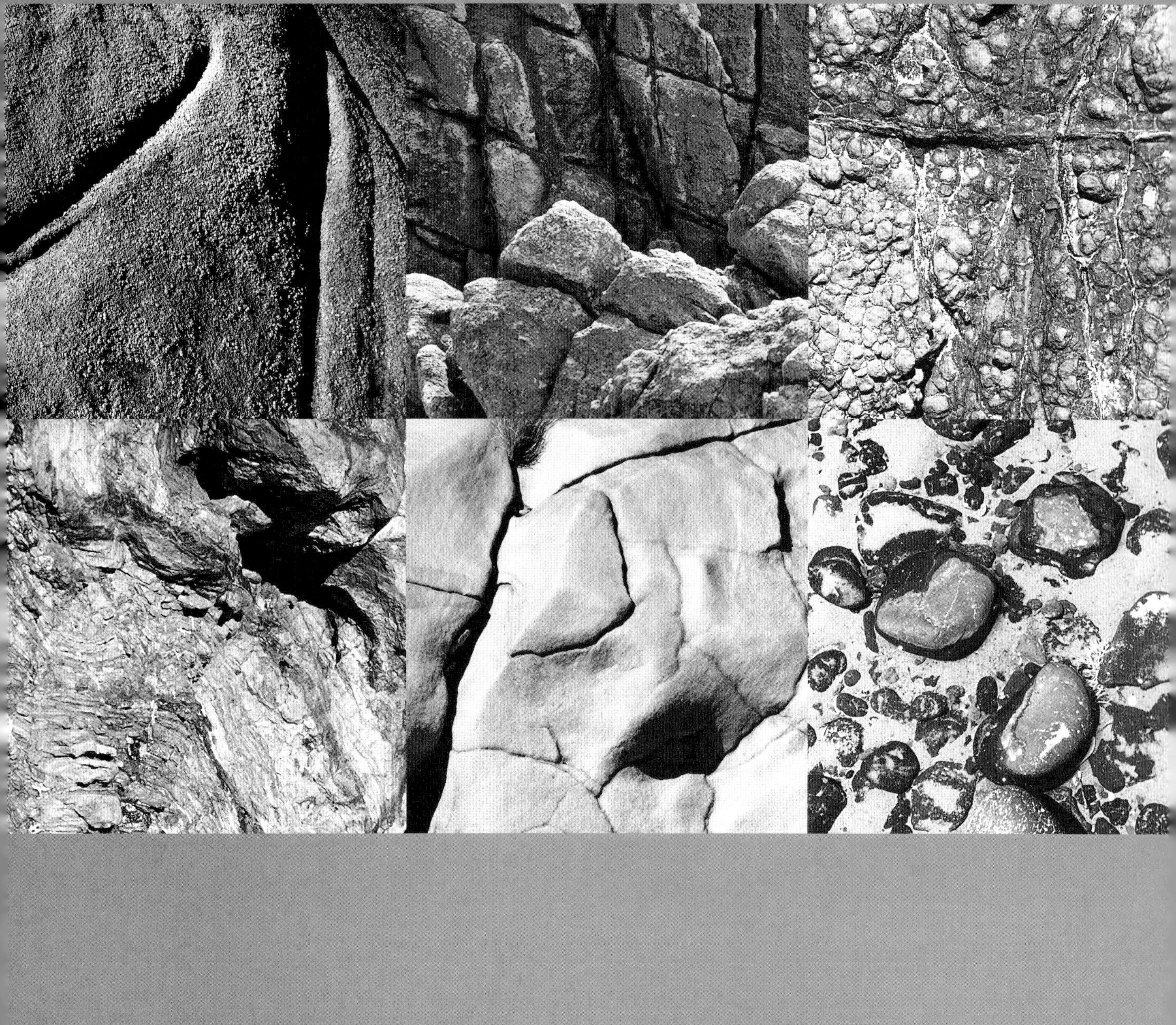

Grief

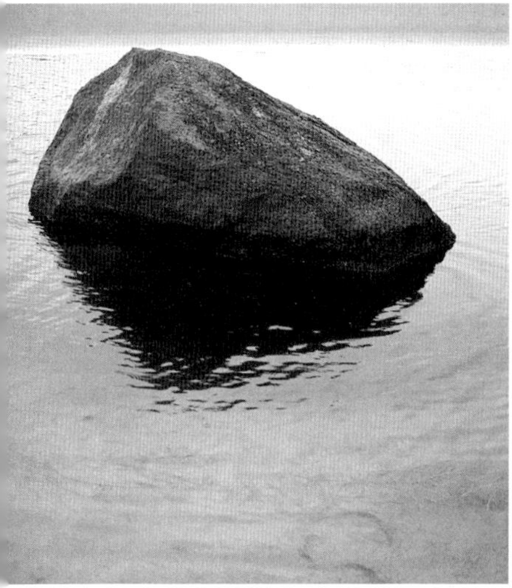

When the Metal element imbalances we feel grief, or grief imbalances the Metal element, depending on how events occur. Traditionally, grief and the act of sobbing is associated with the Metal element and in particular with *lung* channel energy. The Metal element sets boundaries and therefore gives us an understanding of personal loss. When we lose someone we love our body may hunch at the chest and turn inward on the lungs. Our breath carries the sounds of weeping and our inspiration is segmented by the breaks in the rhythm of our breath. Our desire to accept pure Metal Qi through the intake of air is disrupted and we may lose the will to 'take in the world'. We retreat within.

With the coming of the autumn, the season of Metal, we turn away from the yellowed ripeness of Earth and the brilliant reds of Fire's summer. The trees are nearly bare, and the air hints of the chill of winter. The colour of Metal is white; it pales the rouge of blood and brings us closer to things less concerned with fecundity and action. Our spirit stills in silent commune as we begin to turn within.

Grief is a way to reconnect with the spiritual life. We temporarily detach from worldly life; uninterested in seeking pleasures and activities, we seek instead silence and solitude in a quest towards resolve and inner peace. Stillness allows us time to heal and gather strength before moving out into the world again.

Meditation on Metal

Sit comfortably in your meditation posture, your body upright yet relaxed. If you enjoy incense, light some as a gesture of reverence to the cosmic breath, or to your higher self.

In this meditation keep your eyes softly open looking at the ground a few feet ahead of you, and begin to centre yourself with conscious attention and focus on the breath — in and out through the nostrils, your tongue resting lightly on the roof of your mouth.

Breathe deeply into your abdomen, feeling the expansion first in your lower belly and hips before it moves to your chest. As the breath leaves, let it fall from the chest, and then empty from your belly.

Enjoy the space between breaths where no activity is necessary and let your new breath begin again when it naturally will.

Begin to be aware, as you follow the breath, of the underside of your body. Feel your connection with the ground below you and the solidity of your pose.

Feel too the way your head connects you with the world above.

You are grounded, but not compressed. Solid, but permeated by the breath.

You are a rock.

As you breathe, continue to watch the space between the in-breath and the out-breath — so still and quiet, imbued with the harmony of the meeting of the two.

You are a mountain.

From here you can see objectively that the soul world is real. From here you can see that events and phenomena in your physical life are transient. From here you know that each breath brings inspiration and the calmness of connection with your higher self. This is a place of communication that has no words.

Allow your breath to slow and to become very gentle. Close your eyes for a minute before finishing your meditation, and concentrate on the colour white. You may have a beautiful melancholic feeling rise up in your chest.

During the day contemplate the qualities of forgiveness and release.

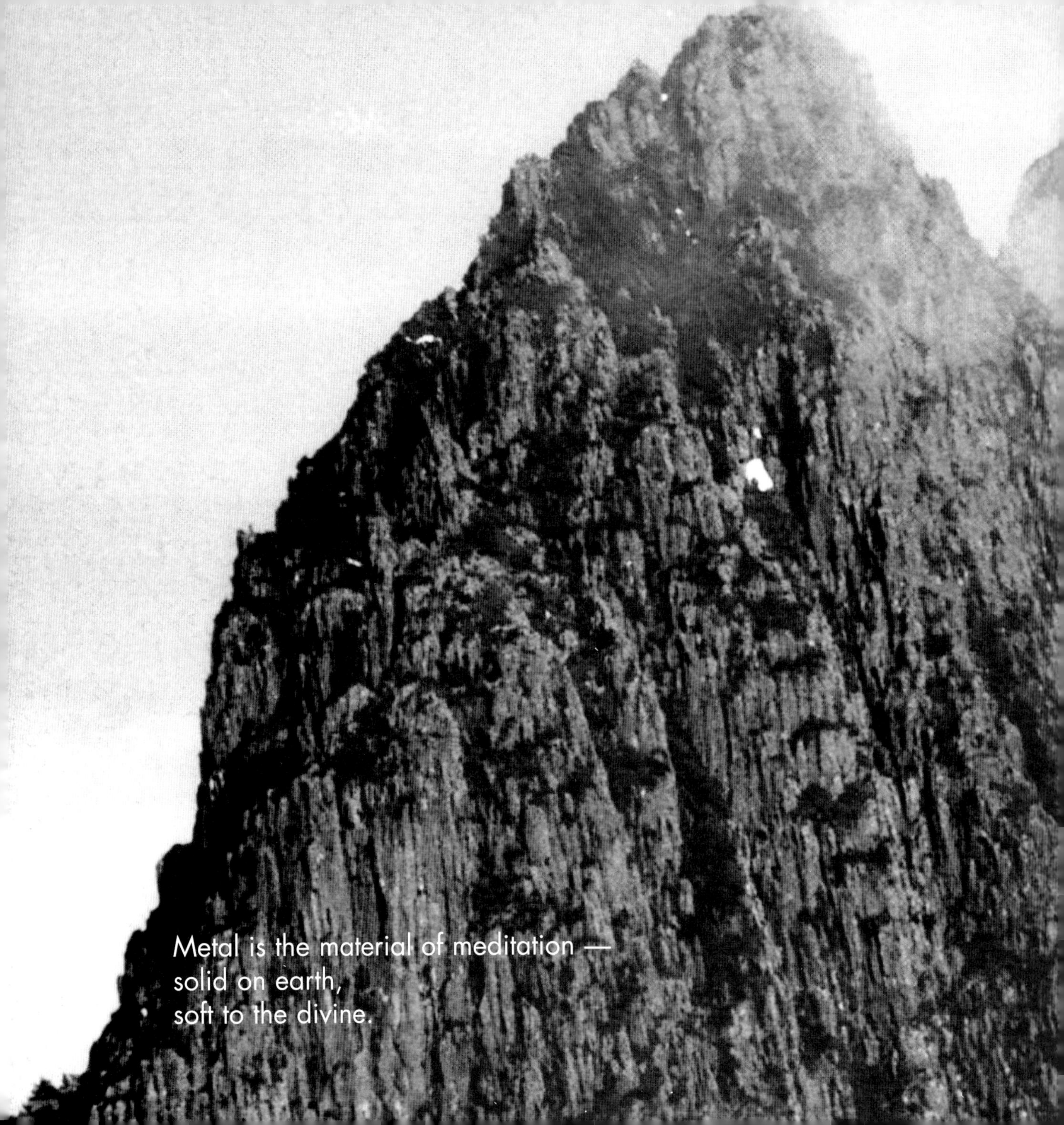
Metal is the material of meditation —
solid on earth,
soft to the divine.

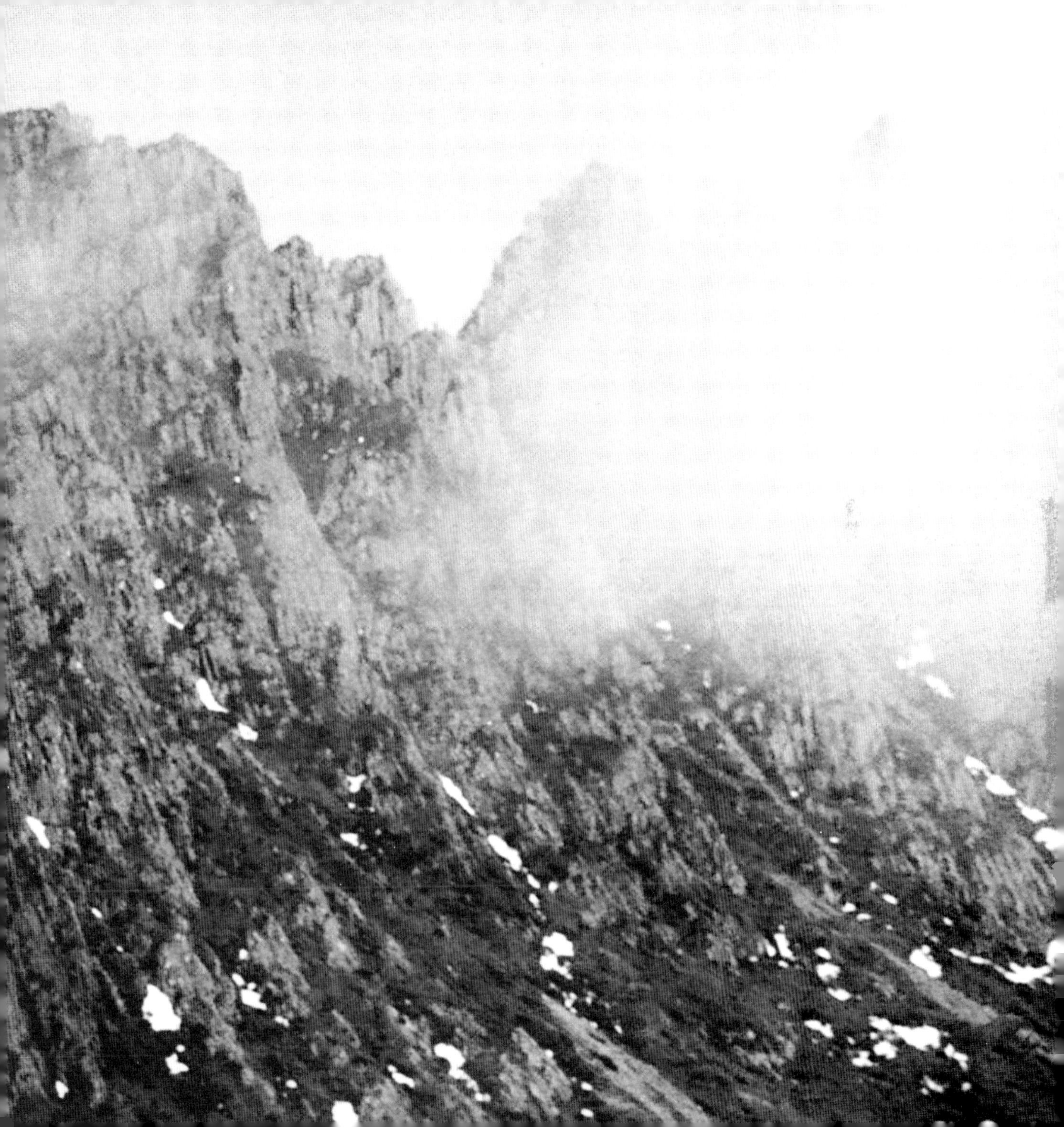

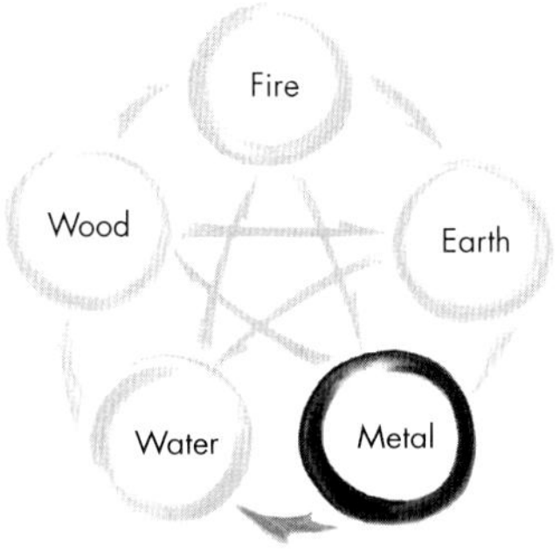

Metal energy in Traditional Chinese Medicine

The Minister of Qi

I am the Minister of Qi and the highest official within the Emperor's circle. I am concerned with the qualities of both inspiration and careful restraint as I exchange the old for the new. Inscrutable, I am a master of discretion and I excel in diplomacy. I am idealistic and the high principles I seek allow me to see the potential in any situation. Through my breath, I am the first contact with the outside world and the last to let it go.

The Metal element channels and important points

In treatment, the channels of the Metal element are largely concerned with disorders of the Qi in the body. These metal channels are named after the organs that most immediately supply and benefit from the Qi that flows in them. They are the *lung* channel and the *large intestine* channel. The *lung* channel begins near the top of the chest and flows down the inside of the arm, ending near the nail of the thumb. The *large intestine* channel begins at the index finger, courses the outside part of the arm and up the neck, and ends near the nose. This channel carries an abundance of Qi.

- *Taiyuan*, meaning 'Great Abyss', is the ninth point on my *lung* channel. As the source point of the lung it has great value in invigorating my energy. It is the Earth point on this channel, where Metal is found, so it is good for all chronic lung problems.

- When I am in the beginning stages of a cold or flu I need *Hegu*, which means 'Joining Valley' because of its location between the thumb and index finger. Fourth on the *large intestine* channel, this point expels Wind from the surface of the body, before it goes deeper. (See 'The climates and the organs' on page 175.)
- If I suffer with a cough or asthma then the right stimulation to *Lieque*, meaning 'Broken Sequence', will help my *lung* Qi descend correctly. It can also assist in overcoming constipation. This point has a connecting channel with *Hegu* and is often used for hayfever or sinus problems. *Lieque* is the seventh point on my *lung* channel.

Metal element channels in the body

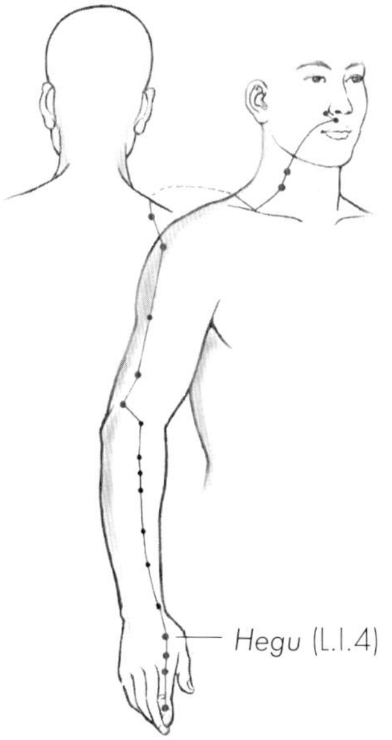

Large Intestine — Yang channel of Metal

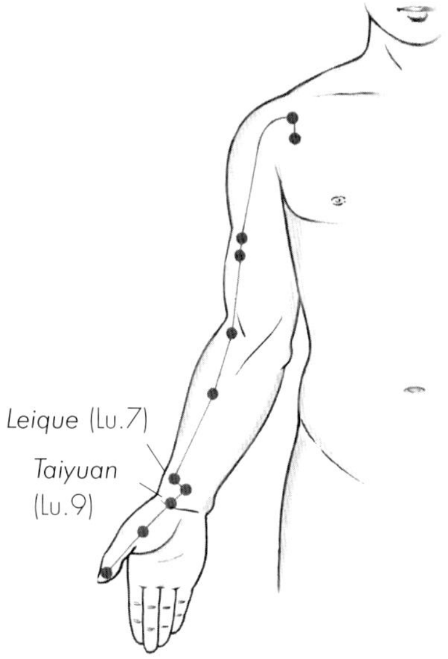

Lung — Yin channel of Metal

The Metal element within our body, mind and emotions

Body

My lungs and large intestine are the coupled organs of the Metal element. In Traditional Chinese Medicine they are responsible for functions beyond the obvious. They are both at the beginning and end of a process; both organs first absorb then release. The direction of my energy is diffused downwards. Cough tells me my Qi is going the wrong way and failing to descend. My lungs produce *Wei Qi*, a defensive energy that forms a protective barrier. Susceptibility to coughs and colds or allergies may mean a distortion or weakness in my Metal element. Treatment of many immune system disorders involves building the strength of *lung* Qi. A weakness can also result in the lungs misreading signals and overreacting to what is normally of no danger, causing allergies to such things as house dust or pollen.

The strength and timbre of my voice depends on the vitality of *lung* Qi. My nose and throat are governed by the Metal element, as is my sense of smell. Asthma tells of *lung* Qi failing to descend. If this is aggravated on exertion, then my *kidney* Qi is failing to reach up to grab my *lung* Qi.

Depression and grief can cause my large intestine to become sluggish. Movement here means letting go; literally and symbolically this means not holding on to the past. Chronic diarrhoea can point to Metal's inability to absorb fluid. My skin is also considered an organ of absorption and excretion and it too comes under the Metal element's control.

Mind

I am like a sculptor's uncarved block or a blank sheet of paper: pliant, sensitive, and open to inspiration. When I cling to outdated ideas there is less room for innovation and I can become pessimistic or lost in nostalgia. I am revived by the optimism of sensing numerous possibilities. As I release the old, my spirit of expectation rises.

Emotions

Grief is my principal emotional challenge. Change of any type requires letting go, so changes always bring a level of associated grief. I may appear preoccupied as I entertain my high ideals or indulge myself in melancholy.

Metal replaces the old with the new,
and inspires objective awareness.

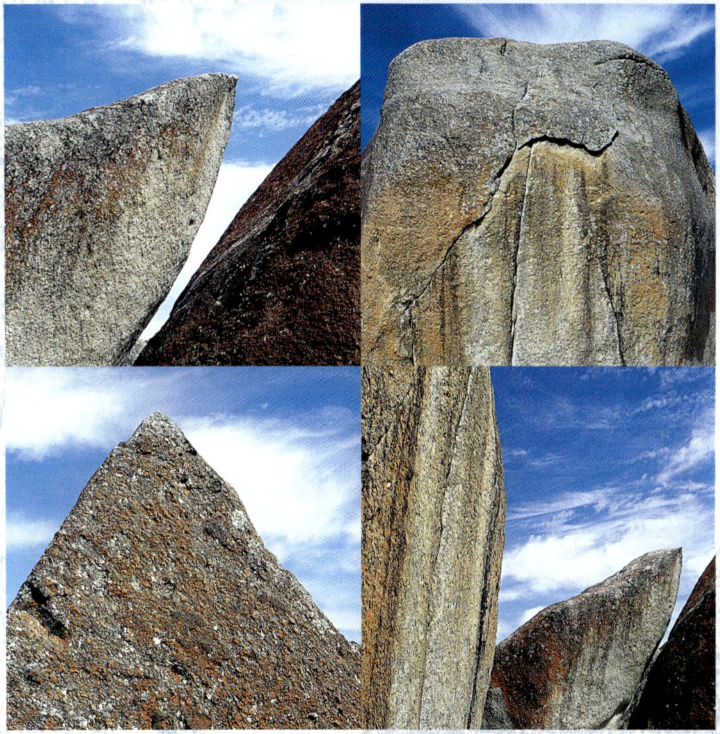

Through release I find fulfilment,
through creating I am created.

When there is weakness in my Metal element the little upsets in life can cause me much grief; the loss of a loved one may be intolerable. In resolving the range of emotions accompanying grief, acceptance replaces loss and I start to move on. I reach this point more quickly if I avoid the temptation of holding on for obsolete reasons. As I cultivate optimism and hope, a sense of amazement invigorates my soul and my ability to cope with change is strengthened.

Destiny of the Metal element

Like a great sculptor, I see the promise and beauty that resides within a block of stone yet to be hewn. Through inspiration, I create through being created. My destiny is to remain in the present, open to new ideas, new adventures and new inspiration. I recognise what cannot be changed and move on with hope and optimism.

Wisdom and age
are the pigments of my pale form.
I condense, become rigid;
yet I am breathing the winds of heaven.

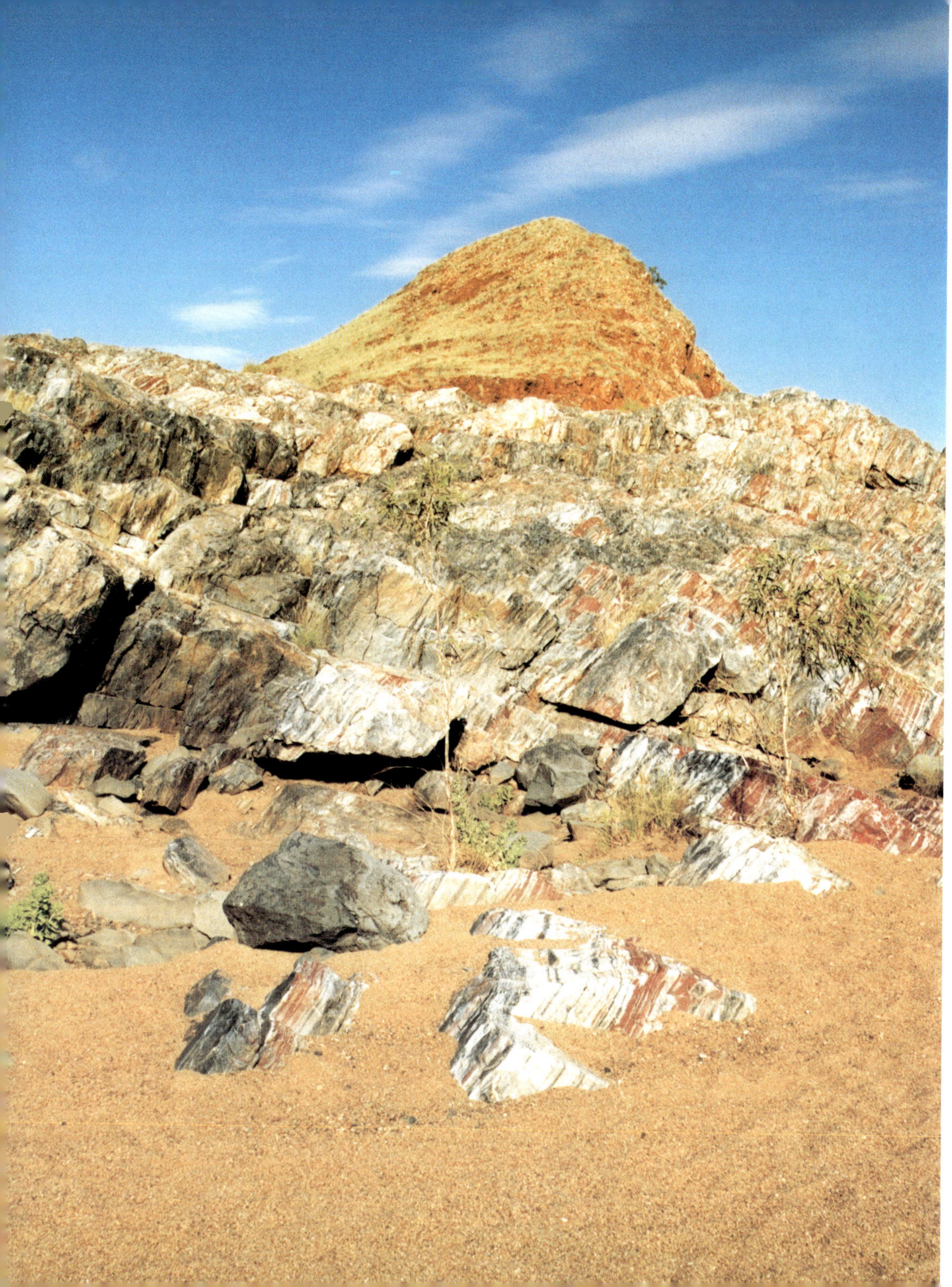

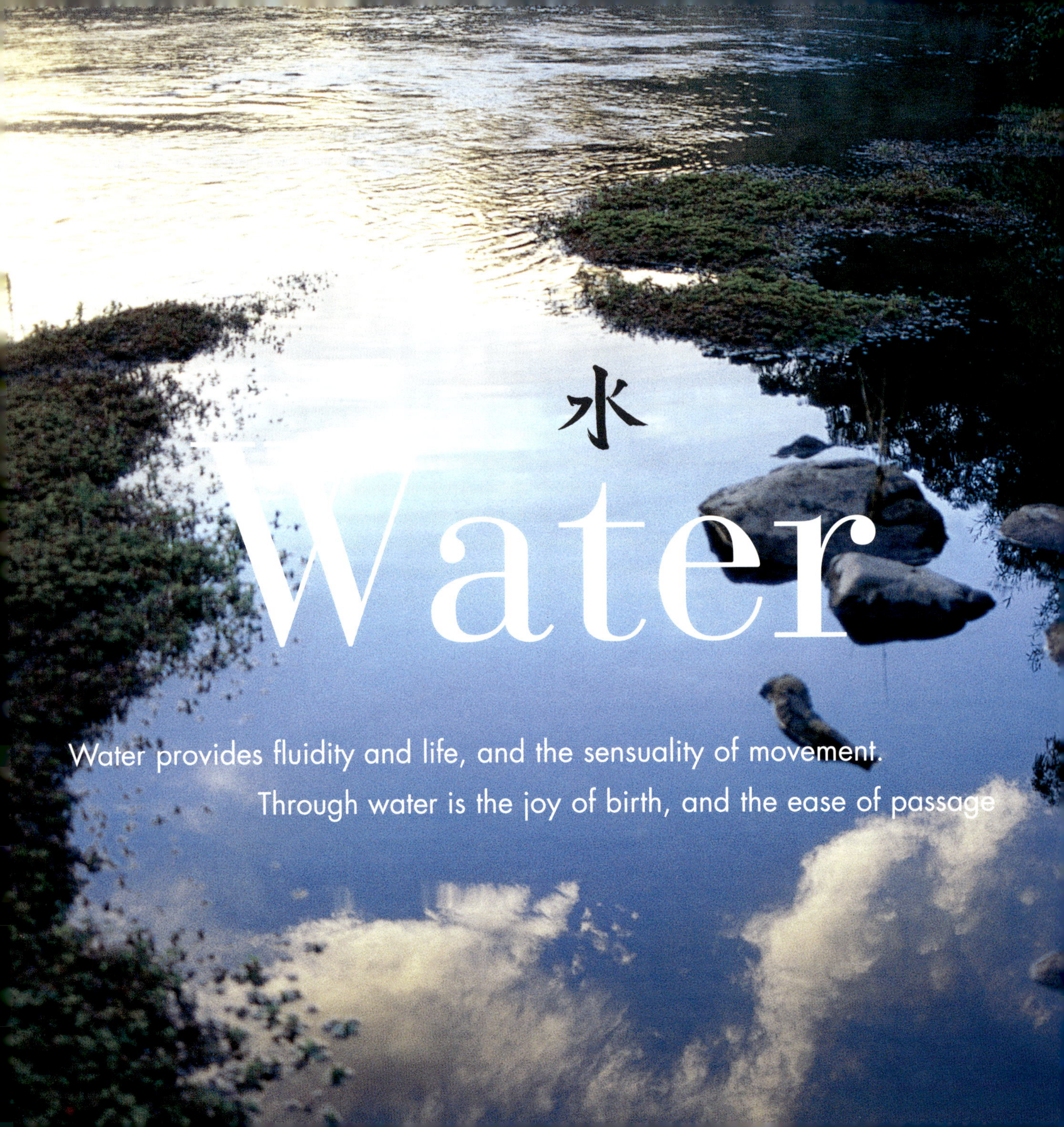

水

Water

Water provides fluidity and life, and the sensuality of movement.
Through water is the joy of birth, and the ease of passage

Water

I am the essence of constant movement —
touched and touching in the
oneness of exchange;
ever adapting.
I am the united body of this stream,
the inherited gift of interaction,
the now moment that
speaks of forever.
You may never touch the same me twice.
I give you flexibility of choice,
the courage of transition,
and interconnection.
I am constant of resolve without any resolution,
Willful of purpose and the right to be;
I am the giver of life;
instinctive.
My body-mind whispers of our destiny.
There is power imbued in softness.
Strength in the non-rigid;
I cannot be broken.
I flow and weave in karmic remembrance:
cyclic, spherical, and pure of form.
I am the embodiment
of active creation.
My nature is forever out-flowing.
I come without language
but will be listened to.
My name is Water.

Traditional Chinese Water element associations:

Winter, black, fear, groaning, the ears, the north, cold, the kidneys, the bladder, the bones, the salty tastes.

The Water element expressed in nature

The Water element manifests physically in rivers, oceans, ice, clouds, rain, steam — and in so many other natural expressions. Water is the elemental symbol for biological life and our vehicle of continual creation. We are completely dependent on the energy and manifestations of the Water element in its many transformations; there is no aspect of earthly biological life that is not permeated by the substance of water, and no physical life can exist without the abiding essence of the Water element. Our very bodies are filled with this mysterious substance; every sense we process delights in its presence. We are visually surrounded by it, we breathe it, feel it move within us, hear it in its many forms and even taste it! Water is life.

Water substance has the ability to change shape to suit any environment; it is never lost, only transformed. It is gaseous when boiled, liquid when temperate and solid when frozen. We witness daily, in the cyclic passage of water substance on earth, this ability to transform: the rain forms streams, runs into rivers, flows into the sea, evaporates, and becomes rain clouds. The clouds empty most of their contents on the high peaks of the land and the cycle continues, all beautifully co-ordinated. This flexibility is the inherent strength of the Water element.

The power of physical water inspires awe. To watch thunderous surf pound the shore fills us with feelings of excitement. Ice and glaciers split apart rocks, falling rain washes away hillsides, geothermal steam blows boulders into the air, and hail stones dent steel! Yet water can also lull us to sleep with a gentle shower on a tin roof, or play with the light to make rainbows.

Our bodies echo the earthly transition of water substance; we have our own network of 'rivers and streams', and constantly interact with water as the basic substance of our being. Every day we are sustained by the passage of water: our life-blood flows only because water penetrates every aspect of our physical self and provides the basic

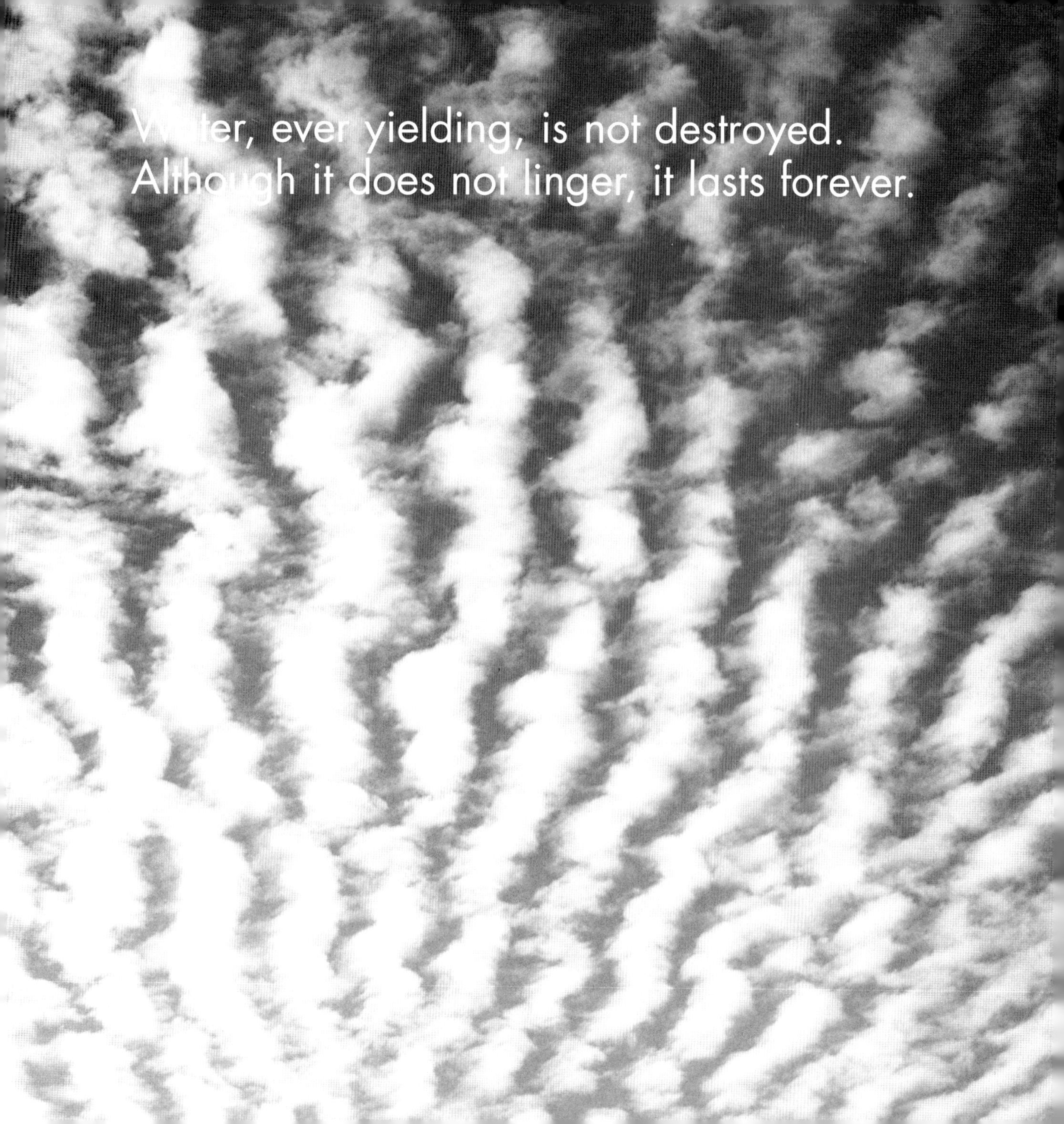

Water, ever yielding, is not destroyed.
Although it does not linger, it lasts forever.

lubrication required for life on earth. Every glass of water we drink has existed for all of creation. It has taken many forms before it became a part of our bodies; it will continue on through us — water is only ever on loan. Even our thinking nature is made up of water. Our brains are 95 per cent water; water allows our thoughts to flow.

Traditionally in Chinese philosophy the Water element is the home of the will — the power of the will to be, to do, to become, to change and to exist. Through the energetic qualities of the Water element we experience motivation. Through our connection with the spirit of the Water element we feel the passage of time and the will to create.

The Water element, the most biologically fundamental of the elements, is the agent that best symbolises constant passage. Water must by nature move. It moves freely in our atmosphere, soaks through the earth, pumps through the vessels of plants and circulates in the bodies of animals, connecting all life with the fundamental gift of motion. In the human body there are no fixed forms and everything is in a constant state of fluid transition. We are like a whirlpool on a river: the whirlpool continues to exist as a form, yet the water that shapes the form is transient and constantly renewed. An exchange takes place at the point where the form appears; there is a constant flow of Qi circulating within the form. As we grow old our body loses the ability to allow this passage and our Qi diminishes. We start to literally 'dry out' until eventually we 'return to dust': we are devoid of water. The water has now continued its wondrous passage and lends its life-giving qualities to new forms; like a river it flows ever onwards towards its destiny. The old saying 'you cannot stand in the same river twice' reminds us of the nature of impermanence and the joy of movement and change — the joy of the Water element.

The primeval or primordial pool is symbolism for the life-giving forces of the Water element. Biological life stems from amorphous water — from the 'collective unconsciousness' of the pool. In traditional Five Element theory, Water energy occupies the space between life and death; it is concerned with the movement from one to the other. Although it is the medium and conveyor of life, Water energy requires a spark from fire before it can create physical life forms. When there is no warmth, water remains as solid as ice or as black as the unfathomed pool.

The river speaks a love letter,
written in the rain,
carried by the mountain,
longing for the sea.

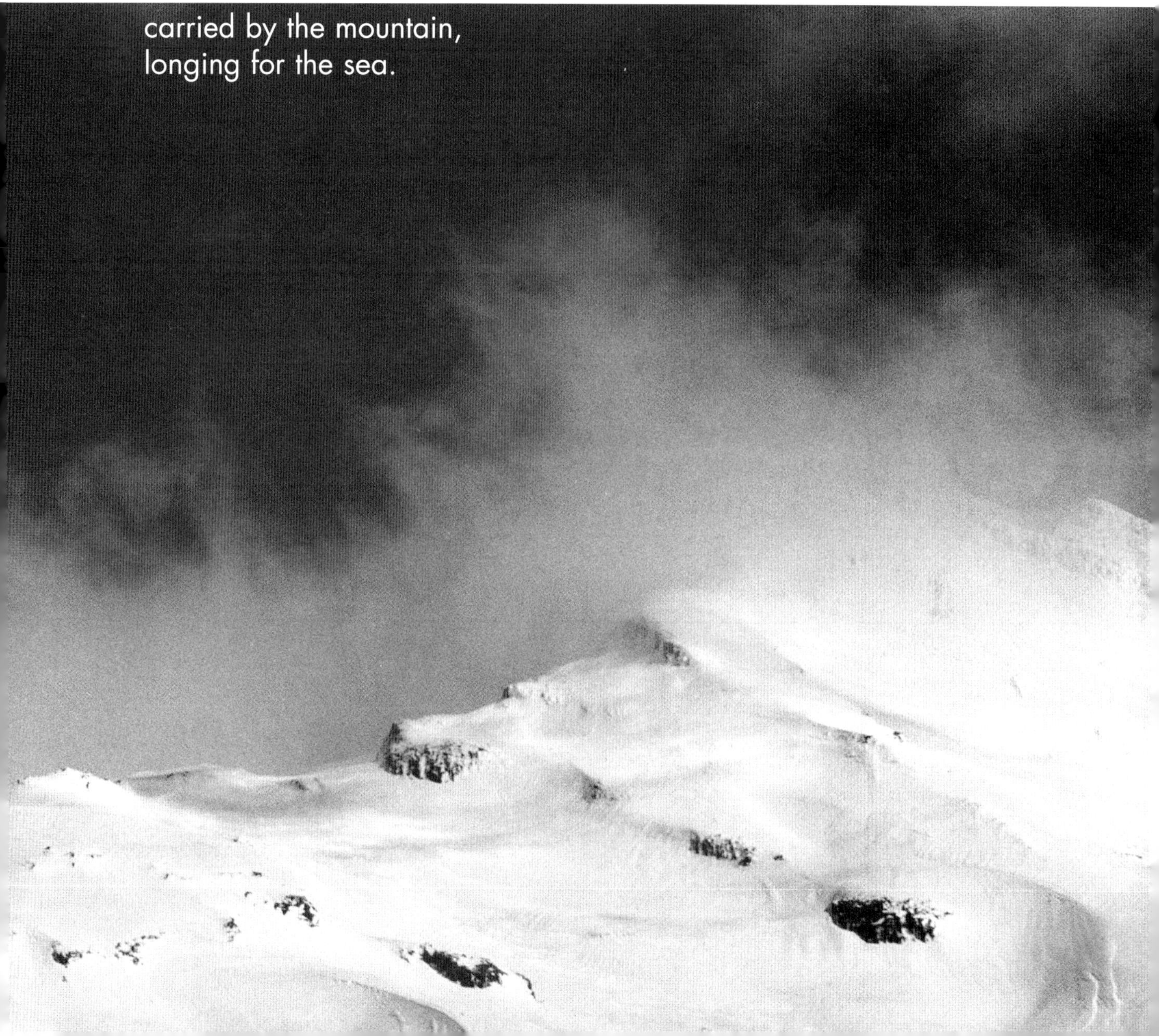

Sacred Water

From the holy River Ganges to the baptismal font, most cultures identify with the purifying powers of water through the act of immersion. There is a sense of return, of rebirth, of putting aside our earthly concerns and committing ourselves to the divine; the weight of human heaviness is washed away. Even the simple act of taking a bath seems to cleanse our mind and spirit. Water touches our very soul and soothes our world-weary bodies.

In many creation myths water is present before the act of the world's creation even begins. Water is the material from which creation is initiated, before life itself is inspired by the event of light or the breath of the winds. In evolutionist theories the earth rises up from the waters and creatures begin to emerge onto the land. In cultural practices around the world we revere the qualities of the Water element with natural symbolism and sacred objects.

The river travels ever onward in an embodiment of the qualities of constant passage. Through immersion in this body of water we receive the gift of renewal; our past is carried from us and we are renewed. In most cultures rivers are sacred.

The fountain symbolises life and our love of movement. We use the fountain as a gathering place … a community focal point of beauty where we can acknowledge the abundant gifts of life-giving water (the fountain of life!) and enjoy the perpetuity of cyclic harmony.

The font holds the symbolic power of water to free us of our misgivings and impurities. Through compassion we are cleansed and are able to move forward, offering compassion to others. We cleanse ourselves in order that we may commune with the divine.

The ocean symbolically represents the great body of the eternal oneness from which we originate and to which we will return. In an attempt to understand its nature, the Dao is sometimes likened to an ocean, the great source.

The rain cleanses the Earth and initiates fertility. Rain is the fertile Earth's lover; it brings the promise of new life, the gifts of the Water element. Traditionally the Water element is the creator of the Wood element, which manifests itself in flora.

Birth and inherited Qi

The power of women to give birth is an aspect of the life-giving forces of the Water element. Bodies are built from fluid in a beautiful continuation of life, demonstrating the miracle of the will to live. As a foetus we develop in a world of embryonic fluid, kept safe as we build our earthly bodies. We prepare for the relative separation of independent life that occurs when our mother's waters break. Water is the original and innermost element of our physical being, while the other elements bring us the form, structure and stature of our being. Traditionally, reproductive disorders may indicate imbalance in the Water element.

In the *kidney* channel and organ (the Yin organ of the Water element) we see the role of Water energy as the purifier and controller of 'passage'. Constant passage is important in the kidneys, both physically and metaphysically; the kidneys are the home of our 'inherited Qi' — the Qi that is ancestral and immediately present before our life begins. The kidneys are the organs linked with the concept of perpetuating ancestral cycles: inherited (*kidney*) Qi is received through our parents and gives us our innate strength.

When we look at a kidney organ, an early foetus and an ear (the ear is the sense organ of Water in traditional Five Element theory) we see a repeating pattern in the shape. In fact, if we look at a friend's ear upside down we will see a shape that closely resembles a developing foetus. The correlation is not lost on acupuncturists, who can treat specific areas of the body by stimulating the corresponding areas on the ear; this is a science and an art in itself. The kidneys are particularly supported by treatment of the ear, and a strengthened Water element in a mother is very helpful to a developing foetus.

Water whispers of birth,
of emergence and transition.
Water is the vehicle of inherited Qi:
our innermost will to live.

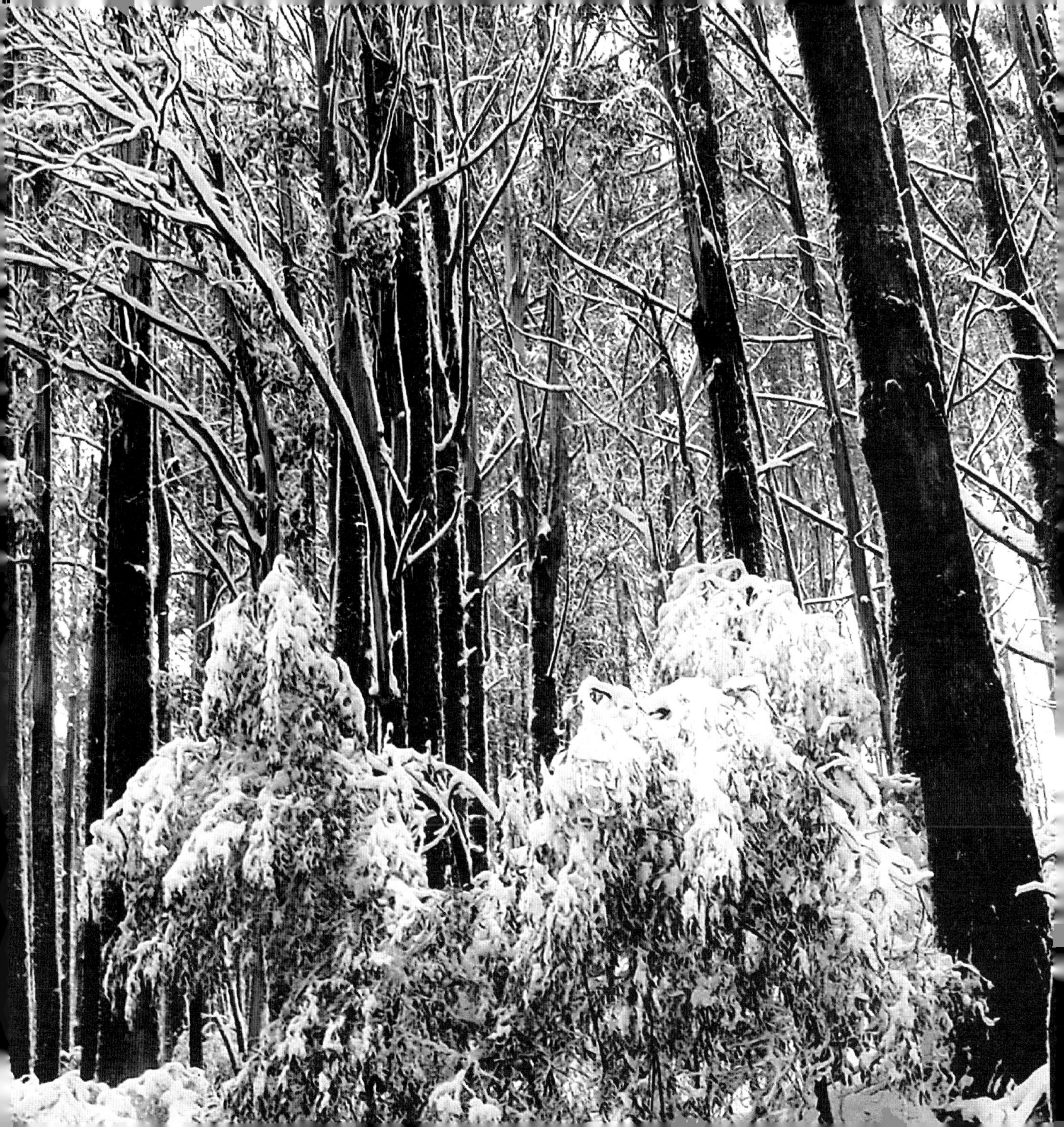

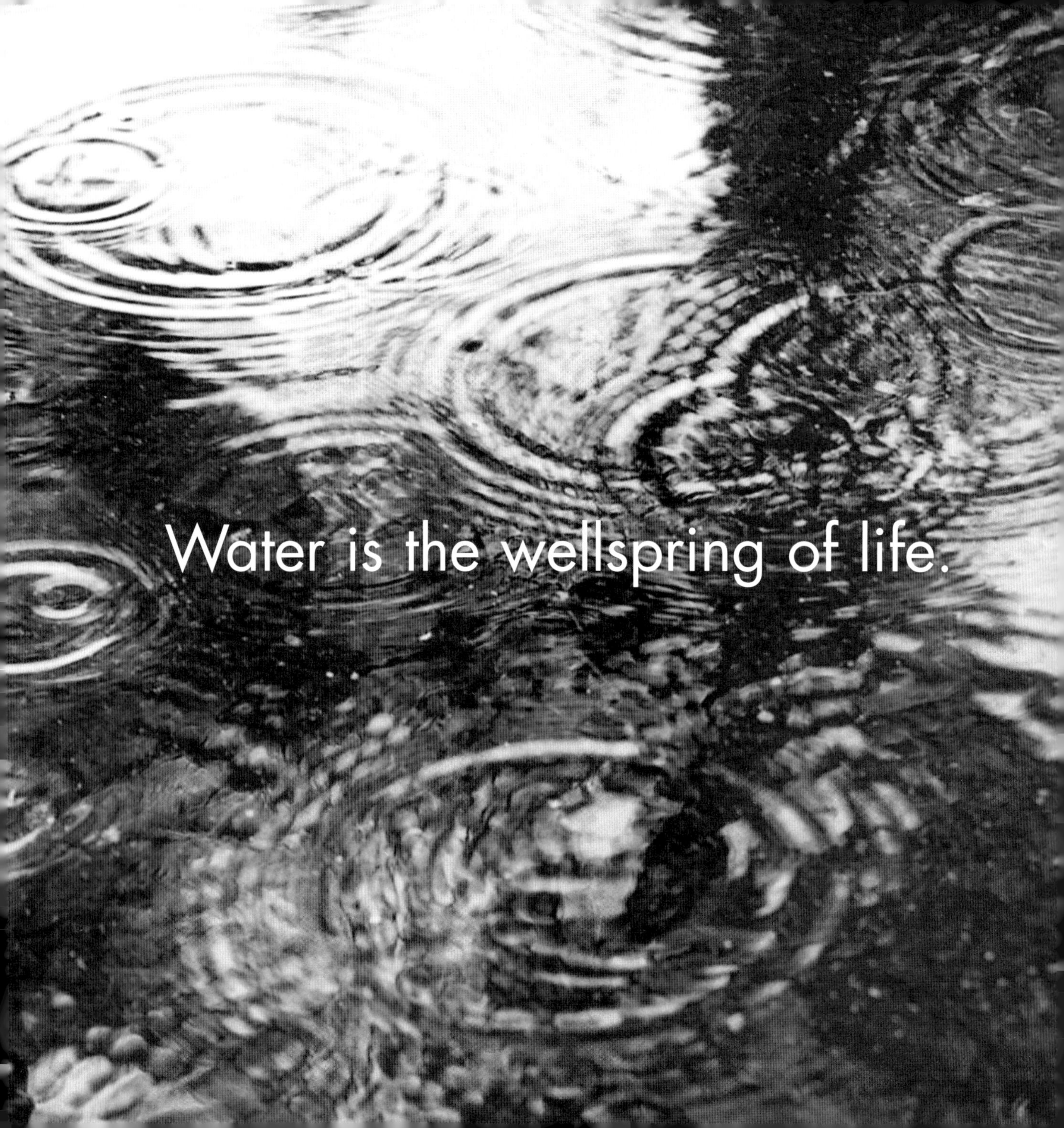
Water is the wellspring of life.

Moving on

A Water element imbalance will often show as an inability to change or an inability to 'move on' with our lives. The energetic qualities of the Water element allow us the softness and rawness of being non-rigid. When the Water element within us is healthy we experience flexibility and have the courage to continually make conscious choices.

The substance of Water embodies through containment and can be captured, but without movement it quickly sours. A 'body' of water loses its life-giving attributes if held in place by stifling forces: life moves on, and so must water. Traditionally the Earth element controls the Water element in the Five Element system by damming it or by creating silt.

Carrying unresolved past issues is detrimental to experiencing Water energy. We clear away the residue and debris of the past in order that we may fulfil our destinies. Sometimes we need to ask the question, 'Past, why do you follow me?' By addressing the past we set the debris free and flow is restored. In that moment we realise that the past no longer exists and that all we ever have is 'now'. This is the great lesson of the Water element.

If our Water energy is blocked we may become fiery in our obsession with the future, but unable to move freely towards this future. We may begin to groan (the traditional sound of the Water element) and complain; we feel too much solidity of presence and have lost our connection with the fluidity of our nature.

Fear, the primordial emotion, is the emotional challenge of the Water element in Traditional Chinese Medicine. Water conjures images of unknown depths and the darkness of a world beyond light and colour. Through selfless love we move away from fear. In being sympathetic and empathetic we transform the fear into love towards others. We become a vessel that allows this flow.

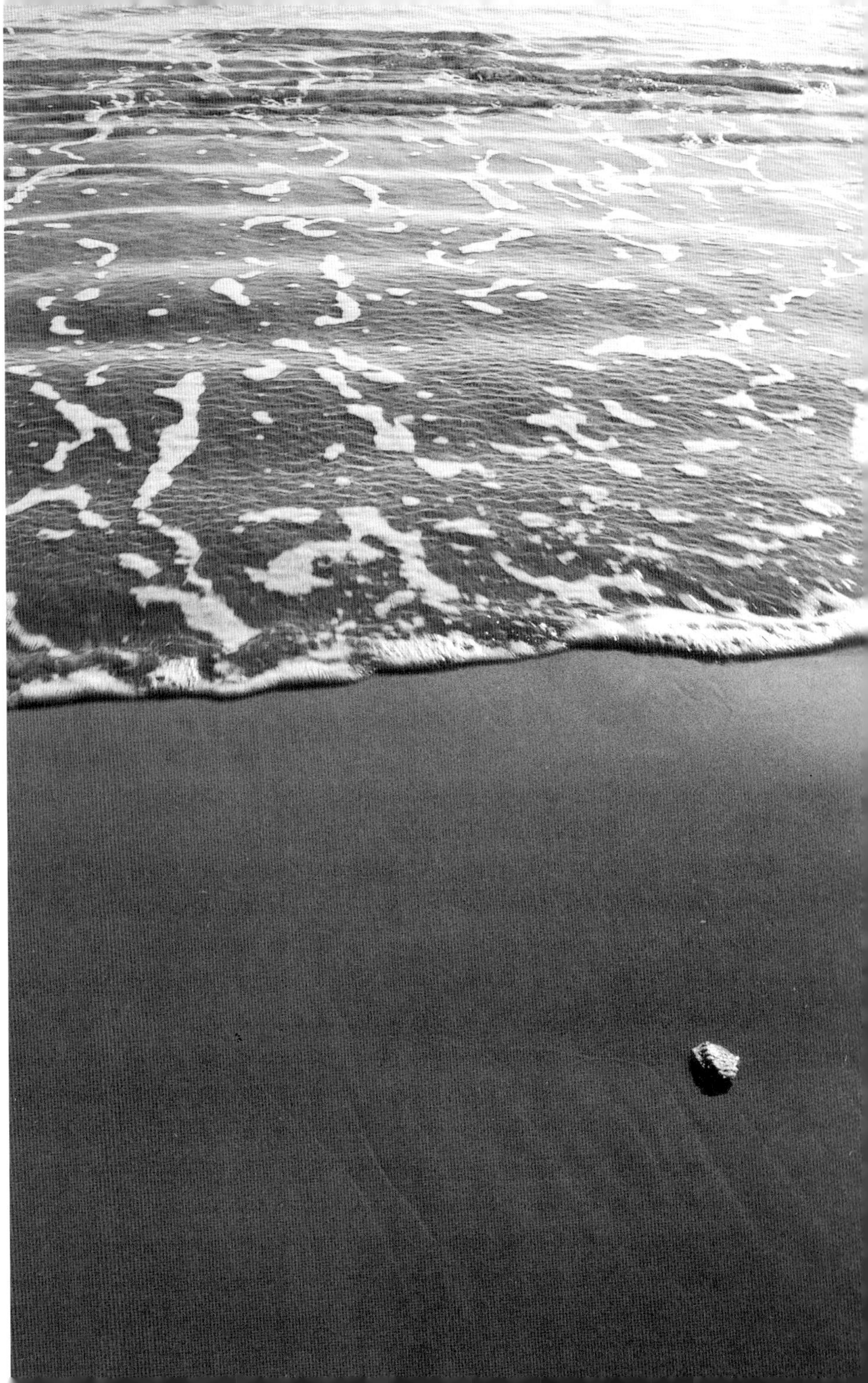

Meditation on Water

Let your body and mind come to rest in this moment and in this place. Sit comfortably in your meditation posture.

Bring your attention to your breathing and watch your breath as it moves in and out of the body, and allow a visualisation to gently guide this breath: as you breathe in and feel the expansion of your belly, have the image of a swell on an ocean rising and building. As you let go of the breath imagine the swell breaking into a wave that rolls across a pebbled beach.

Breathe in through the nose and out through the mouth. The sounds you naturally make echo the sound of your visualised swell and wave, the sounds of the ocean shore: the in-breath gathers a mountainous swell, the out-breath forms an effortless wave that rolls onto the shore.

Imagine now that the swell and the wave grow.
As you breath in, the swell fills you with pure water. As you breathe out (through the mouth), the water of the wave flows over your body like a cascading fountain of pure clean energy emanating from the crown of your head. Feel a sense of release, as your fears are washed away.

Stay with this image for a time until the breath is fluid and free, rhythmic and steady, like the ocean of your visualisation. When your meditation nears an end, gradually slow the movement of your breath, until your breathing is so gentle it is almost imperceptible. Let your mind come to rest in a deep, still pool. Enjoy the absolute peacefulness of this place.

During the day contemplate the word 'release' and the virtue of courage.

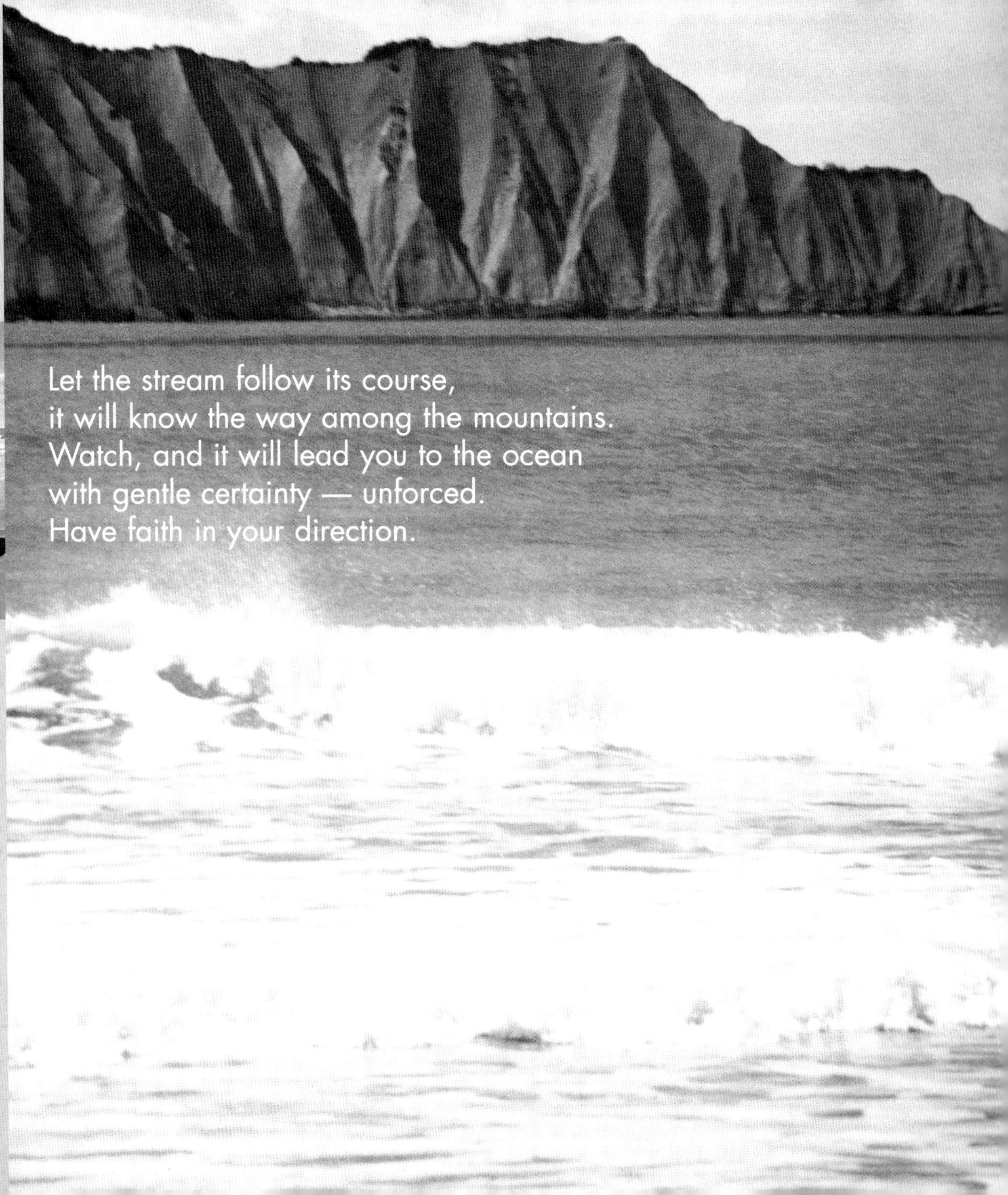

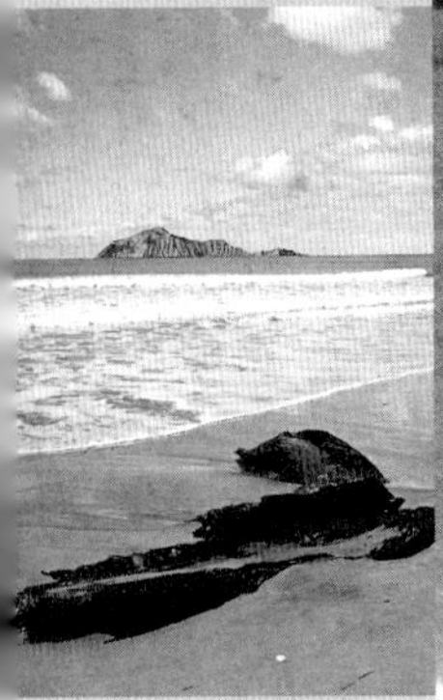

Let the stream follow its course,
it will know the way among the mountains.
Watch, and it will lead you to the ocean
with gentle certainty — unforced.
Have faith in your direction.

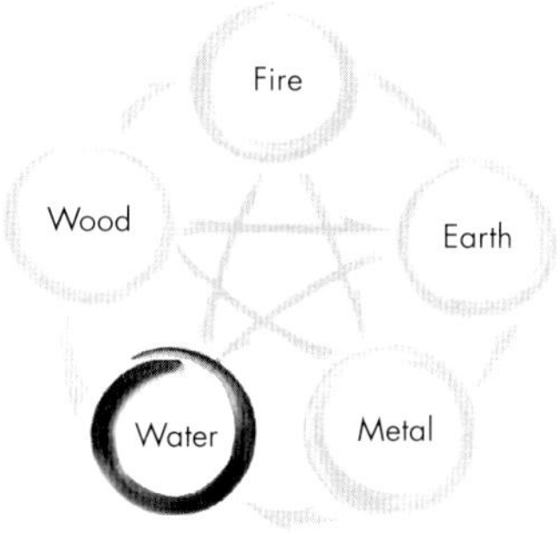

Water energy in Traditional Chinese Medicine

The Minister of Health

I am the Minister charged with maintaining the health of the nation; my role is to balance the forces of Yin and Yang. I am at the root of the body's energy source and I am the gate of life. I contain the knowledge necessary to create life, govern growth and perpetuate the image of my ancestors. I house the will, which provides the plan for my bodily structure and my ability to function on earth.

The Water element channels and important points

The channels of the Water element are important in giving strength to the legs, back and urogenital system. Both of the Water element channels begin or end on the feet, and are named after the organs that most immediately express the Water element's activity in the body: *bladder* and *kidney*. The *kidney* channel starts under my foot, flows along the inside of my leg and over my abdomen, and finishes in my chest. The *bladder* channel begins at the corner of my eye, travels over my head and down my back and legs, and finishes at the nail of my little toe.

- With a sore lower back or a loss of sexual desire I will need *Shenshu*, meaning 'Kidney Transport'. This is the twenty-third point on the *bladder* channel. It will nourish my kidney organs directly and help me absorb the energy from my lungs. It will also assist in building up my stress tolerance levels.

- If I am weakened to my core with a chronic illness or prolonged stress, I can call upon *Taixi*, meaning 'Greater Stream', to help regain my strength. I can tap into the roots of my ancestral Qi through this point and build my essential energies.
- If my memory starts to fail or I have suffered long with a chronic illness, *Gaohuangshu* will work to raise my spirit, clear my mind and help restore memory. It is the forty-third point on the *bladder* channel and is used for psycho-spiritual disorders as well as chronic lung problems.

Water element channels in the body

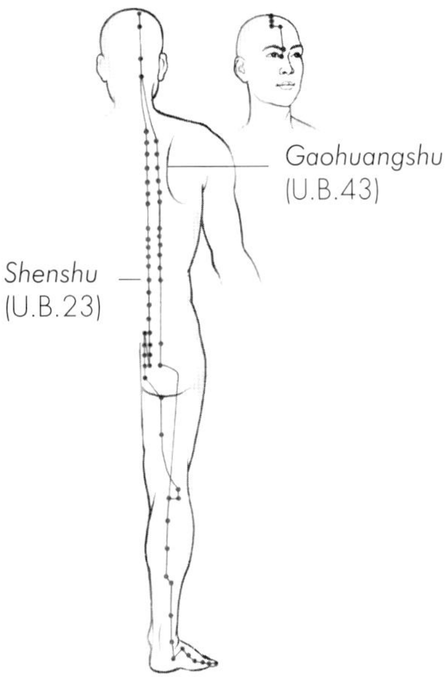

Urinary Bladder — Yang channel of Water

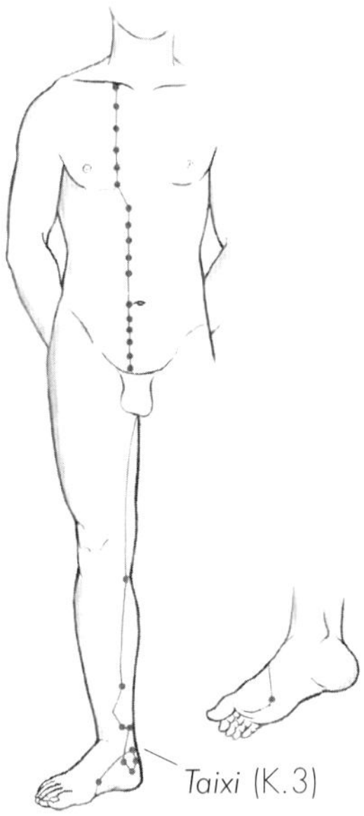

Kidney — Yin channel of Water

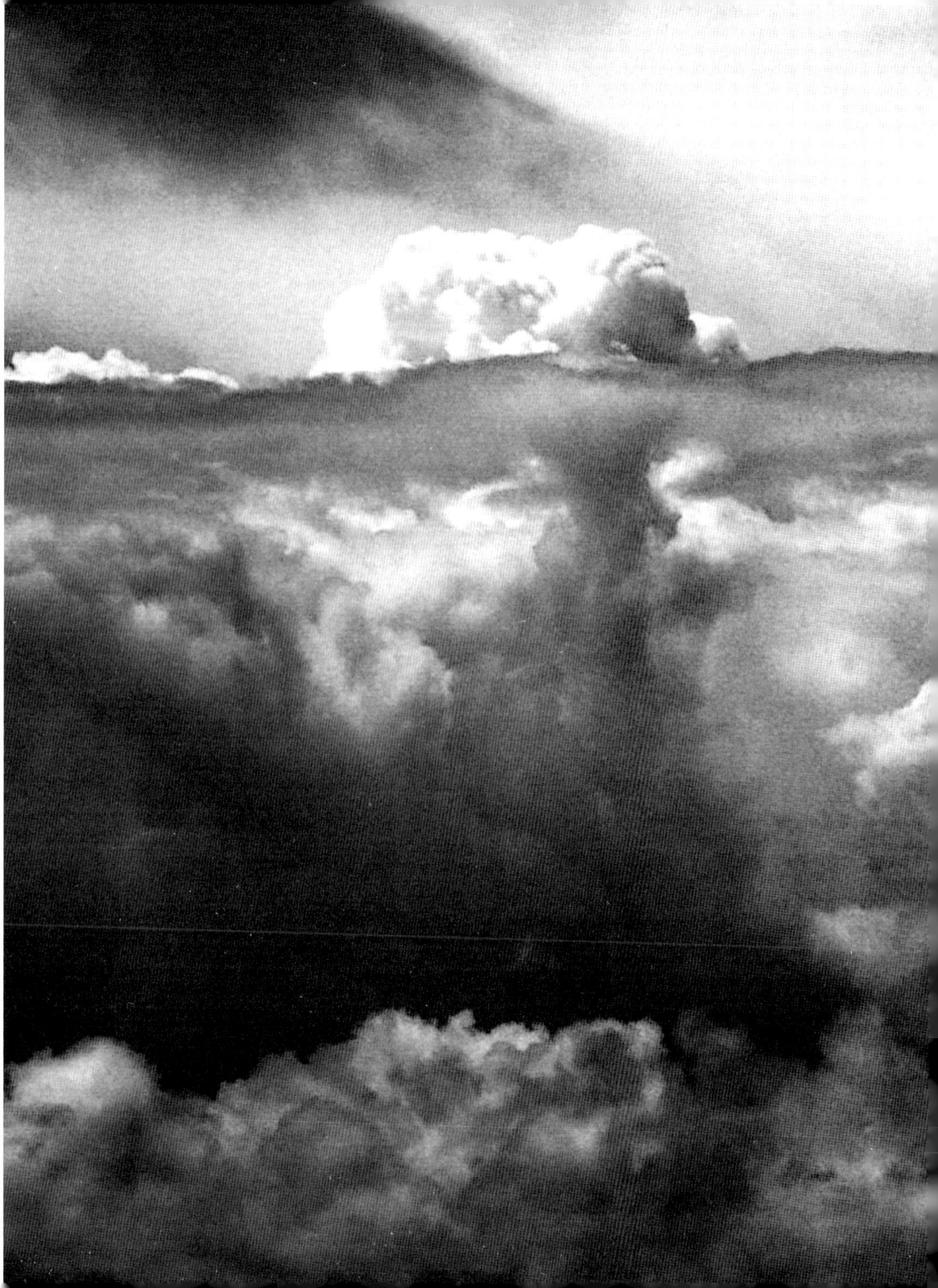

The Water element within our body, mind and emotions

Mind

I govern the mind and all memory resides within me. Intelligent and resolute, I seek challenges that hone my willpower and galvanise my intent. When my reserves are diminished my intentions become diluted and I can give up easily. I become 'wishy-washy'. When I am determined, a strong intent translates readily into action.

Emotions

Fear is the emotional challenge of my Water element. I strengthen my will by meeting each new challenge with courage. Courage contains a seed of fear, and fear is part of courage's virtue. Fear both restrains and activates response and is vital for its ability to put me totally into the present moment. It is fear that awakens my ability to respond with all my senses.

I can be both tranquil and still, or turbulent and full of fright. Fear of the future (anxiety) and fear of the past (guilt) can unnecessarily tax my Water element. Overwork or chronic illnesses can also deplete my vital essence and leave me easily frightened. When I am restored, I am calm and determined; much of what I do is accomplished easily and gracefully, with plenty of energy kept in reserve.

Body

My Water element contains my ancestral memories and provides the genetic blueprint for the shape and form I take. This ancestral Qi is blended with extracts received from the other elements, creating special essences that are stored deep within my body and are circulated as required. My Water element governs growth and reproduction; it nourishes the innermost structures of my being, including my bones.

My ears and sense of hearing are under the direct control of my Water element. Ringing in my ears and any loss of hearing points to an imbalance, as does thinning of my bones and arthritis.

Fluids are regulated in my body primarily by my Water element. In Traditional Chinese Medicine the paired organ of the kidneys is the bladder, which stores waste fluid garnered from the activities of the kidneys. Frequent clear urine can indicate the presence of cold, which can injure my body: the kidneys respond by removing the

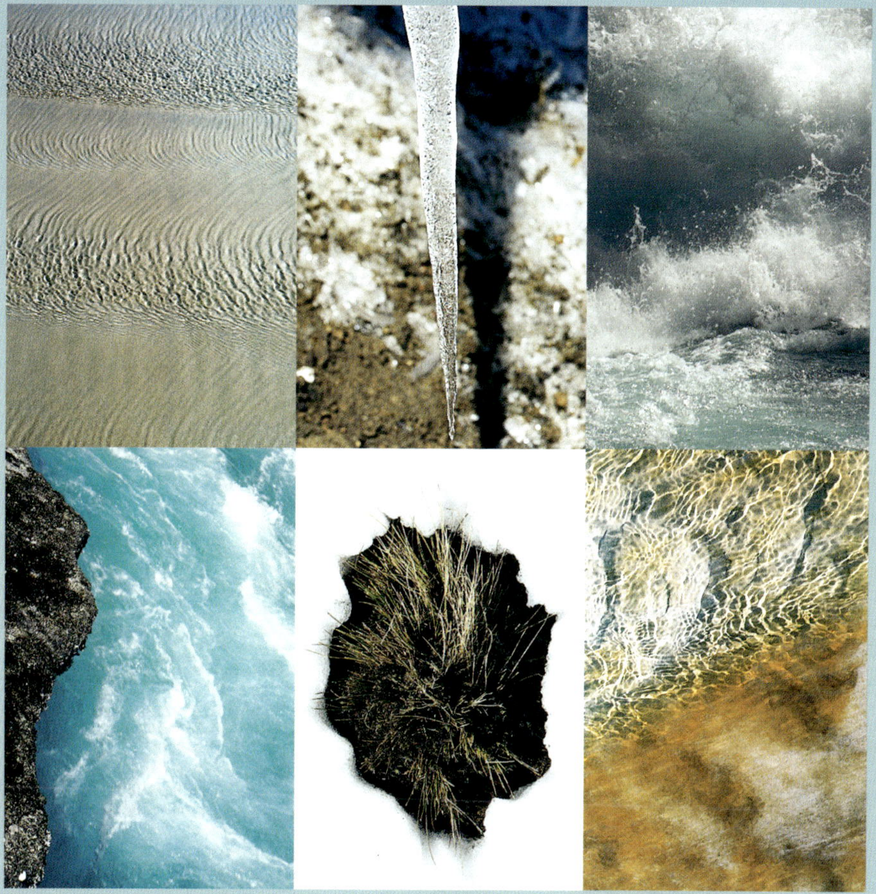

‘coolant’. Alternatively, the presence of scanty darker urine shows that the *Kidney* channel is conserving fluid because of the presence of excess heat.

The strength of my *kidney* Qi reflects into the lower part of my body, especially the lower back and knees. Lower back pain often indicates problems with *kidney* energy. My *kidney* Qi is also responsible for the strength of my hair, while it is *lung* Qi that governs its sheen. Greying and premature ageing is a sign of diminishing *kidney* Qi, as growth is governed by kidney essence.

My reproductive organs are regulated by my Water element, and a strong desire to procreate can mean that the *kidney* Qi is either abundant or affected by an imbalance of heat. The waning of sexual desire as I get older corresponds to the natural depletion of kidney energy. Both sexual excess and lack of sexual expression — according to my age — have important health implications. Excessive sexual activity may drain my kidney essence, while lack of sexual expression may indicate that my Water element needs support. I can choose to conserve the life-giving qualities of my kidney essence and can channel this energy into other creative directions such as art or meditation.

Destiny of the Water element

As the roots of the physical body, my destiny is to provide stability and strength. With my mind I project a clear intention and a powerful will. Through the virtues of courage and composure, I transform fear into determination; so I create equilibrium between the elements. I am tranquil, gentle and self-assured.

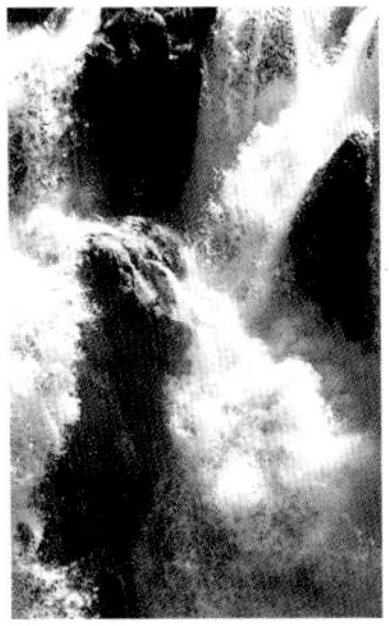

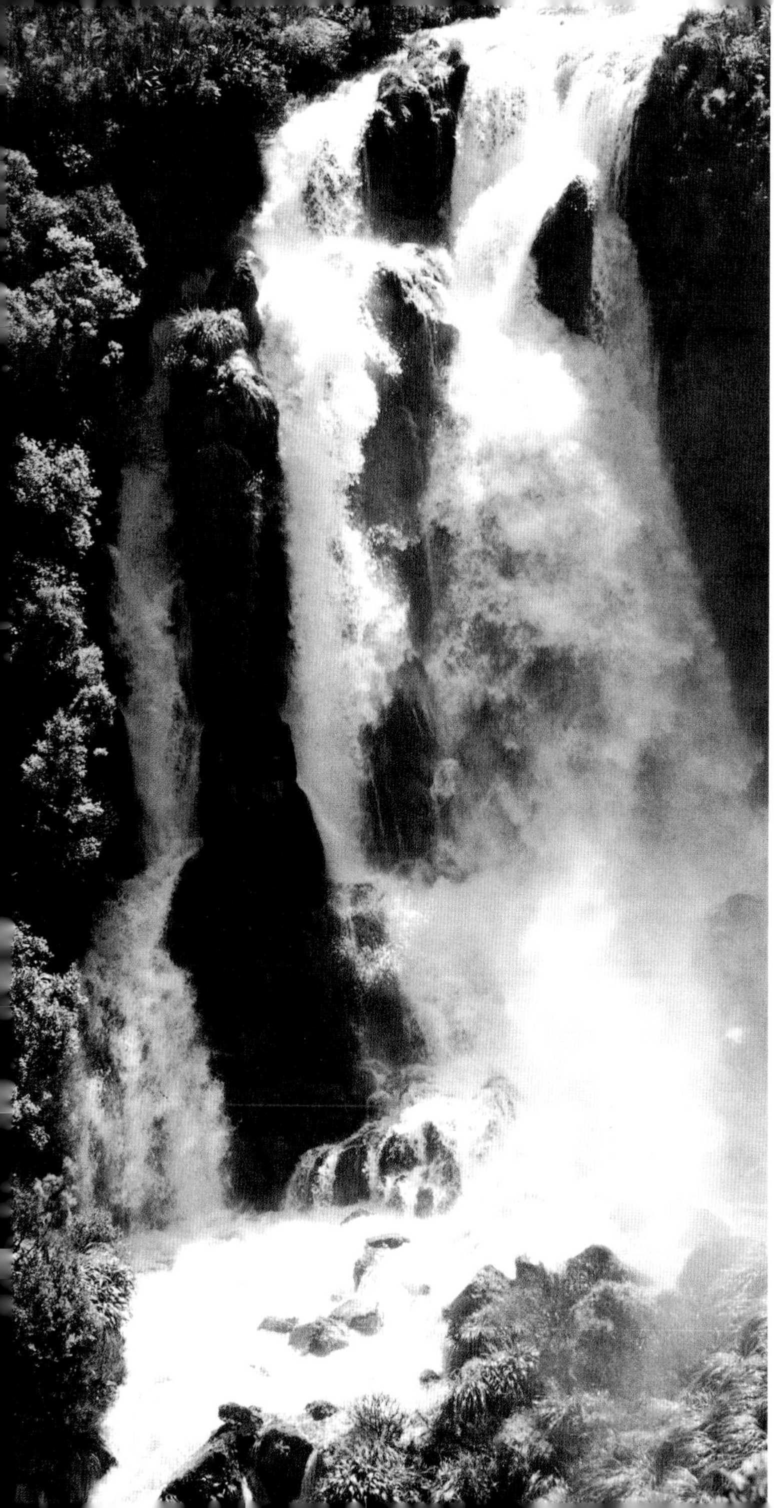

From a single tear,
to a raging storm.
Rain, wash me to your ocean.

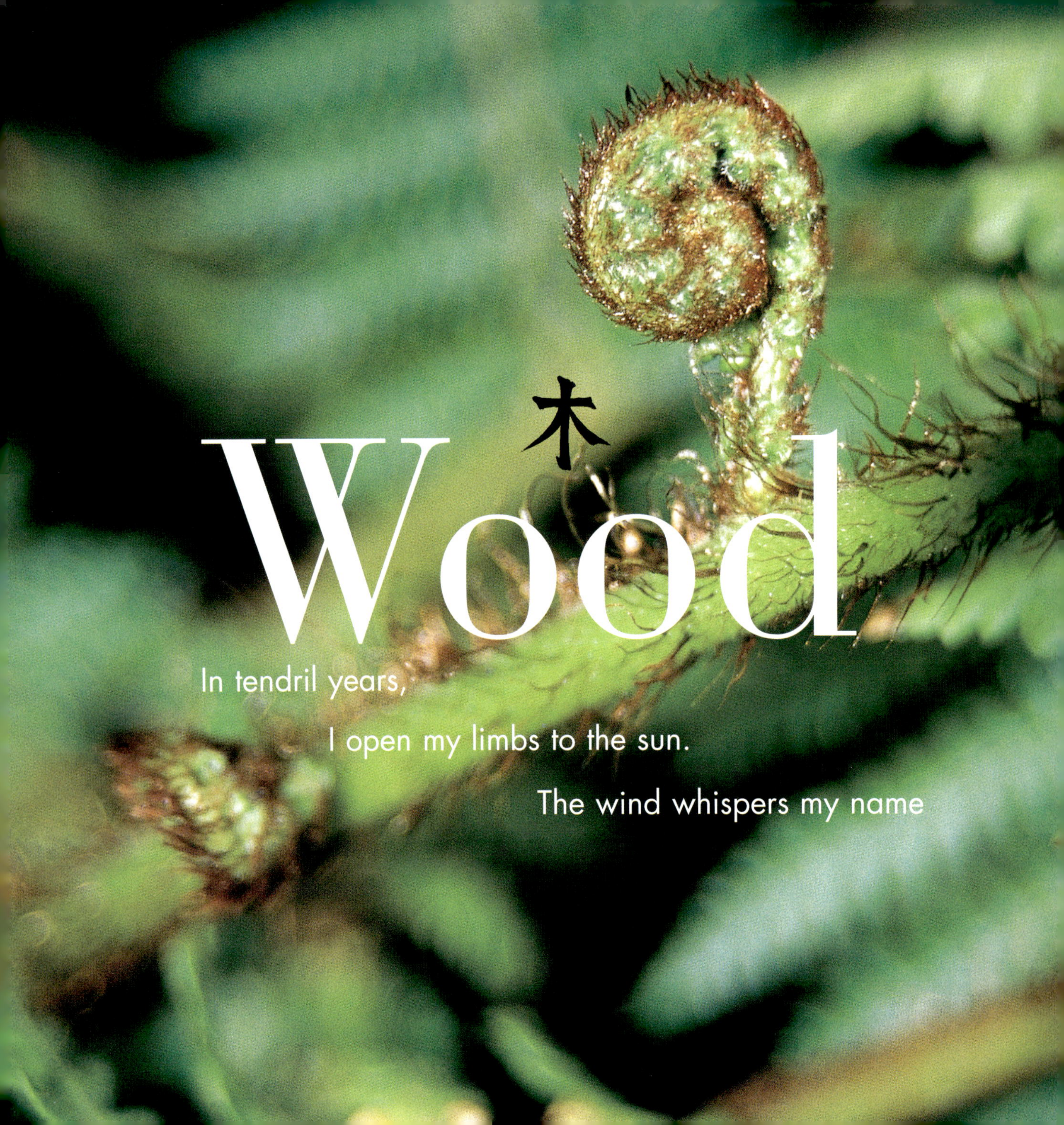

木

Wood

In tendril years,

I open my limbs to the sun.

The wind whispers my name

Wood

I am a statement of being.
I mark this moment and acknowledge my existence within it.
I am actual, decisively present,
building my organs
into organisation.
My structure is mighty, but supple.
At once I plunge deep roots into the earth,
while my tendril green head whispers to my friend the wind.
Formation becomes conformation by my hand!
I will have order!
I will guard this soul.
From this tower I see clearly that my limbs are not unplanned.
I know myself well, and have boundaries
best respected.
I bring the forces of heaven and earth together in my being,
and I speak of new beginnings,
of harmony,
and of striving.
I am ever watchful — unafraid to shout as I unravel the dormant seed.
I am the essence of Wood.

Traditional Chinese Wood element associations:

Spring, green, shouting, anger, the direction east, wind, the eyes, the gall bladder, the liver, the tendons, the sour tastes.

The Wood element expressed in nature

Spring is the season of the Wood element. Nature is exploding into life. As the earth warms, the seeds that held tight over the winter reach out towards the sun like opening arms that welcome embrace. These seeds contain everything required as a blueprint for the plant; they are the message capsules from a past life that will inspire another generation. This is the time of rebirth and continuation of natural order.

The most iconic and powerful expression of the Wood element in nature is a growing tree. A tree stands majestically in a statement of 'I am', growing another ring each year as the trunk reaches ever upwards to the sky. The tree roots burrow deep into the ground to draw the strength to stand tall, to stand one's ground. The branches and leaves of the canopy are supple, flexing in the winds; rigidity would mean weakness. The greenery sways in controlled surrender. These qualities are reflections on the energetic power of the Wood element.

Traditional Five Element theory recognises the number eight as being associated with Wood energy. Our symbol for eight is also used for infinity, which is the nature of a tree's cyclic life. The tree that bears the seed inevitably decays and returns to the soil, only to nourish another generation as the spring sun again strikes the ground and inspires new growth.

Wood energy is the archetypal organiser. The tree organises many sources of Qi to co-operate within its form. The sun brings life through the leaves (photosynthesis); the soil gifts minerals and stability; the wind loosens the seeds and exfoliates the dead matter; water offers the softness and fluidity essential to life; and the tree itself breathes the waste air of the fauna. But all cycles are reciprocal. In return, the tree holds the soil of the hillside together while keeping down the salt tables in the plains; carbon dioxide is exchanged with oxygen by the flora that forms the lungs of the planet. Moisture is retained by the flora and slowly cycled in an act of distribution,

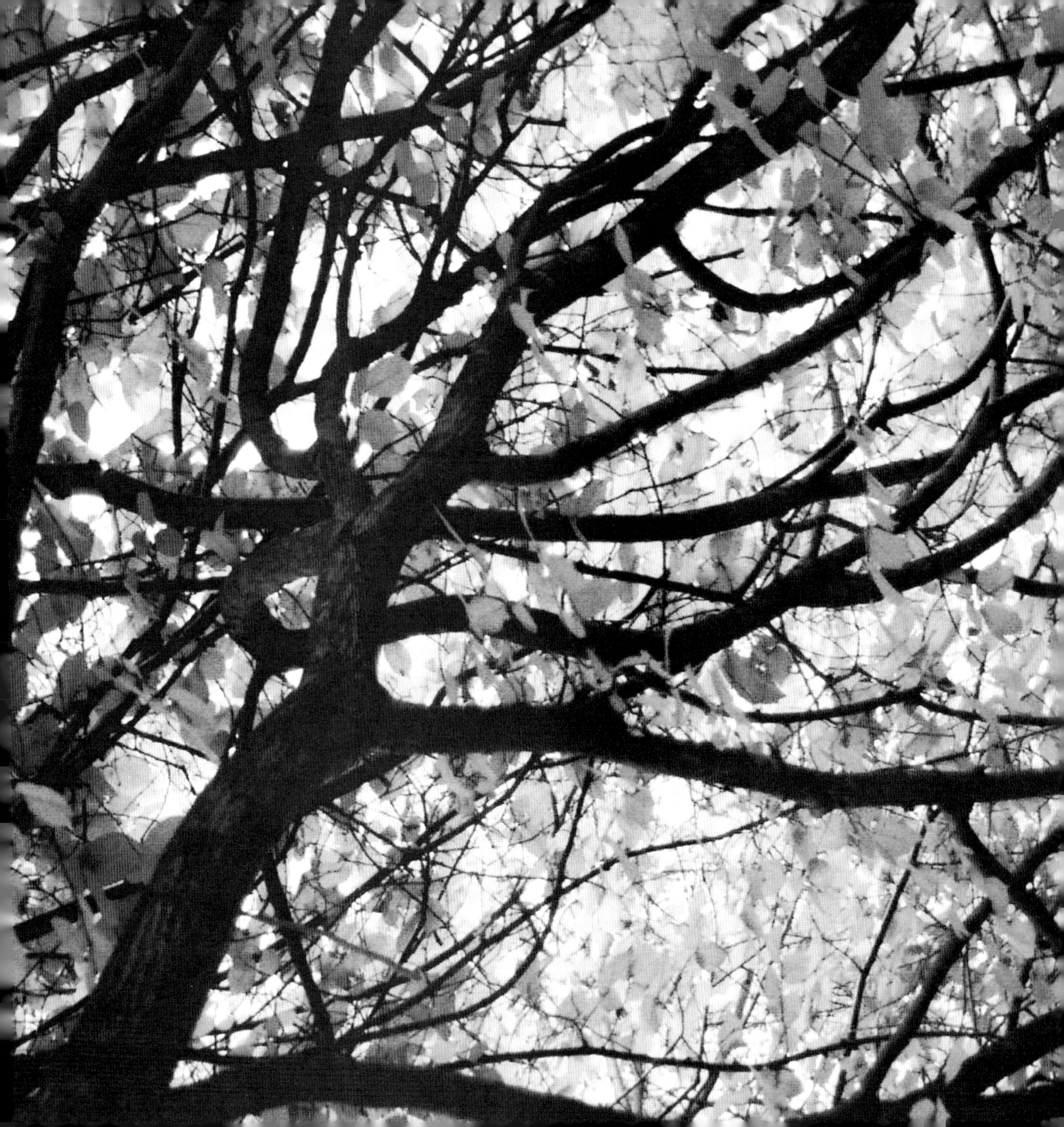

and the body of the tree acts as a sheltering host for other life forms. The Wood element is ever busy in its quest to facilitate and maintain natural harmony.

As treetops bend in the wind, children may be drawn to climb as high as they can go. Children, who are in the Wood-dominant phase of their life (their budding years), love to test their growing bodies by swinging from limb to limb. They are content only when the challenge of the top branches has been surmounted. The energy of the Wood element creates a driving force in our nature; we strive ever onward and upward with a decisive vision of the future. From the heights of a tree a child's view is clear; another generation feels the excitement of seeing a way forward. Our ancestral roots and our own family tree give us the foundation for this journey and for this personal growth.

Spiritually, Wood is recognised as the element that houses the soul. When the soul loses the will to live and is unable to be enthused by the Spring and the joy of rebirth, the body ails. A lost soul will have difficulty being decisive and may feel scattered to the four winds. But when a soul rejoices, decisions become easy, change is a joy, and new beginnings are inevitable!

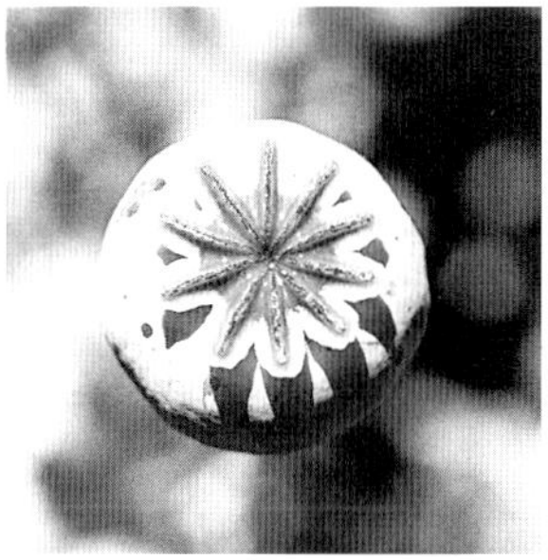

Our soul,
housed by the strength of our Wood,
surrounds itself with the movement of life.

Spring

In the temperate and cooler regions of our planet the Wood element finds its fullest expression in the springtime. This is a time of emergence and movement, and a dynamic force is awakening; it is the early morning after a deep and restful winter sleep. The cello has been replaced by the flute, and the sounds are crisply ordered.

There are many things to be done: it's time to 'spring clean', organise the planting, tidy up the yard, clear away all the cobwebs — so much to do! But not everyone is enjoying this upheaval; the stimulus creates some irritable livers and gall bladders, the traditional organs associated with the Wood element. The wind is the climate controlled by the Wood element, and the winds of spring that clear the sky of impurities also gather around our necks where our *gall bladder* channels are most exposed. People with Wood element imbalances will feel irritable or even very angry; yet these same winds also bring a wonderful clarity to our minds.

Spring is crucial to continuing lifecycles in the natural world, and the strategic energy of the Wood element dominates this season. There is a feeling of purpose in the workings of nature that can be positively aggressive and urgent. Some plants become rampant in their striving; many animals focus all of their strength on vying for the opportunity to mate to create offspring, even if the contest kills them; and many crop farmers take to the fields knowing they must succeed now or lose a year's harvest. Animal farmers will be busy with lambs and calves; orchardists see the blossom and anticipate the fruit season; fishermen in the colder regions paint their boats while looking out to sea; and soldiers begin to march — clad in green, the colour of the Wood element. Everywhere we look we see planning and activity. Our eyes are wide open to our own possibilities, to our earthly responsibilities, to our ability to assert our visions. Decisions are being made and strategies finalised; we are moving towards the future with a feeling of celebration for life. Humans — and nature — aspire.

We tap into our strength,
the deep roots of our nature,
and raise our strong limbs to the world.
Our shoulders carry responsibility —
the ability to respond.
We know what must be done.

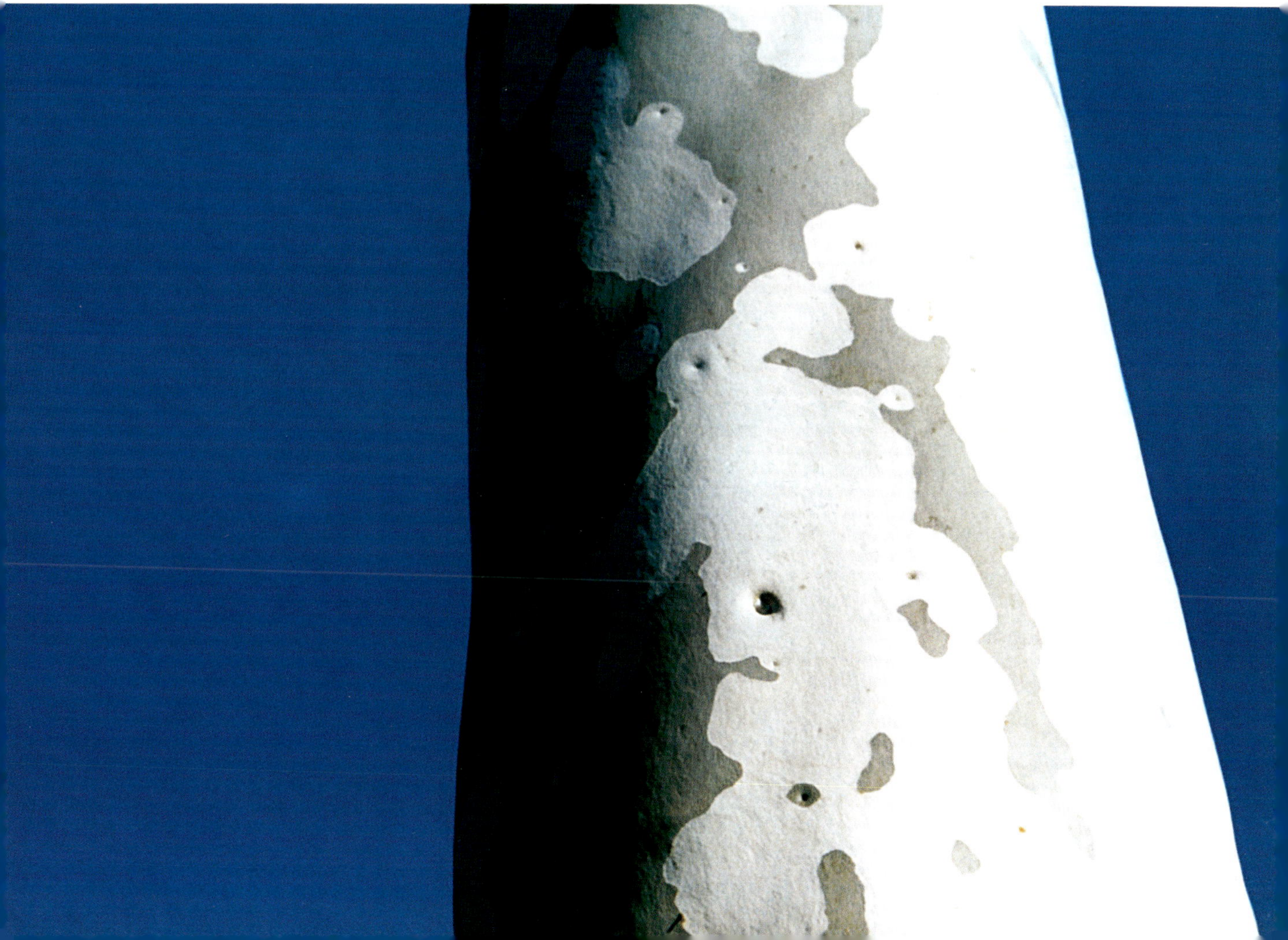

Wood teaches of growth
and the aspiration of ideals.

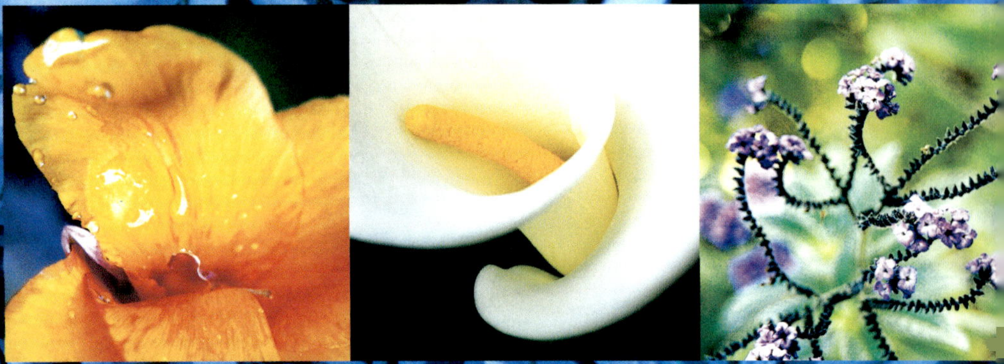

The winds of change

Change is in the air; the sails fill and carry us to new shores. The wind, created by the energy of the Wood element, travels with ease from one place to the next and from one state to the next. We can enjoy the gentle whisper of a breeze, or shout into the howling gale that screams of need for change. The wind exerts force on the oceans, raising the waves that ensure movement and the clearing of stagnation. But too much and the earth will be eroded, because Wood controls Earth in the control cycle.

The wind travels freely,
a vagabond with great purpose,
visiting all the world.

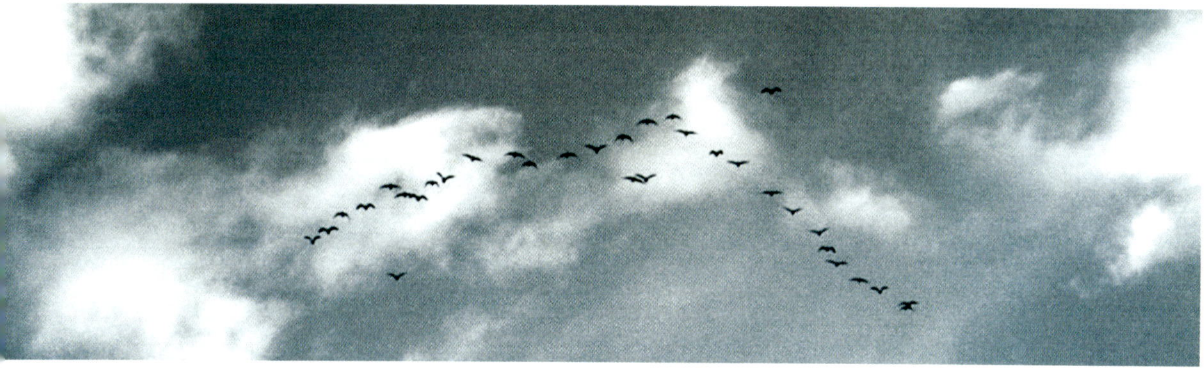

The coming of great events is often heralded in human imagery with the power of great winds. In Christianity the arrival of the Holy Ghost (Pentecost) was accompanied by a powerful howling wind, and the four winds represent the four cardinal points of the heavens. In the Hebrew *Book of Genesis* (*Beresheet*) creation occurs as the winds float on the face of the waters. The wind pre-exists the act of creation, is symbolic of God's breath and is called *Ruah*. In the Hebrew language wind and spirit are the same word. In the Islamic tradition of creation, wind is seen as the agent that maintains order in the cosmos. In traditional Chinese philosophy the Wood element's wind is the great organiser, ever ambitious, seeking order where there is chaos.

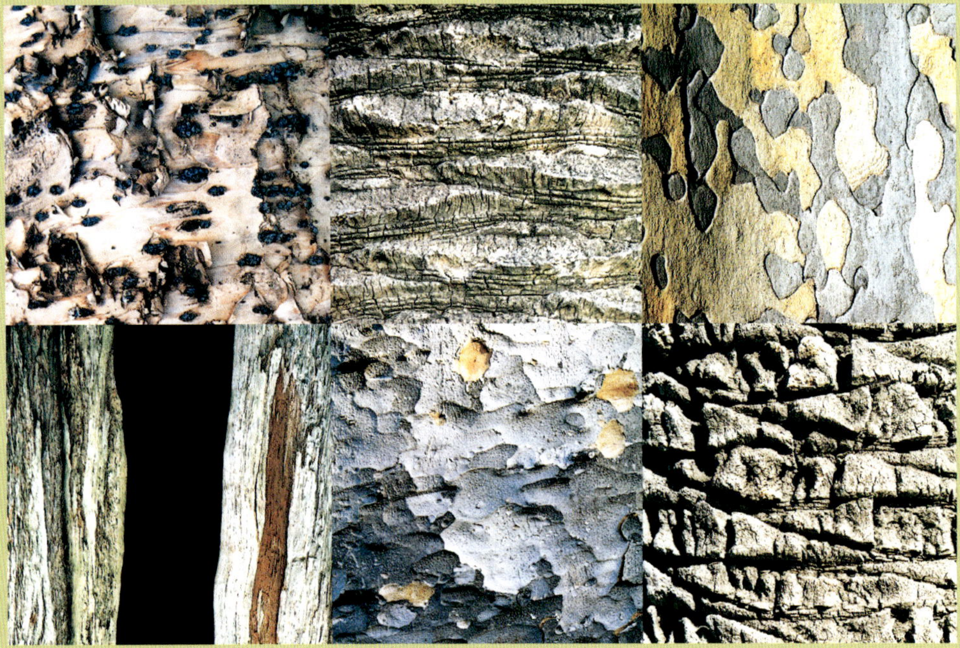

Many cultures revere spirits borne by and of the wind. Spirits are given to move on the winds, as are angels on the wing and the voices of people passed on. Gypsy fortune-tellers are sometimes referred to as the 'mirrors of the winds'. Many cultures also recognise the association of anger with the wind and the ability of strong winds to destroy. In mythology the wrath of deities and gods is often observed in the event of ferocious winds. Anger is the traditional emotional challenge of the Wood element in Chinese philosophy.

When we stand on a beach and face a storm we feel cleansed and refreshed in our soul as we hear the hauntingly beautiful voice of the wind. We feel the power of the Wood element.

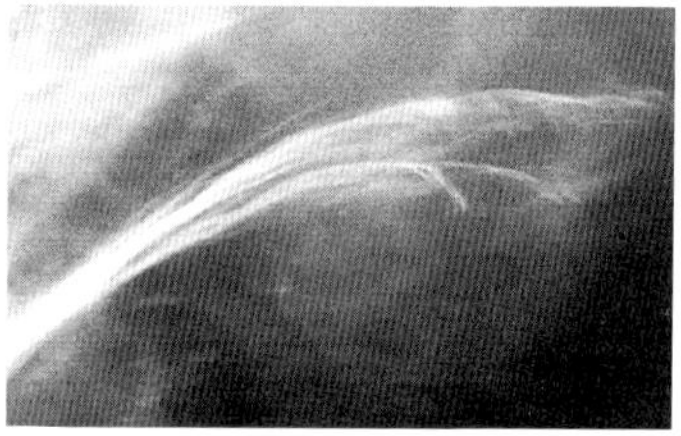

My soulful tears cool the anger of my nature.
I create harmony where there was none.

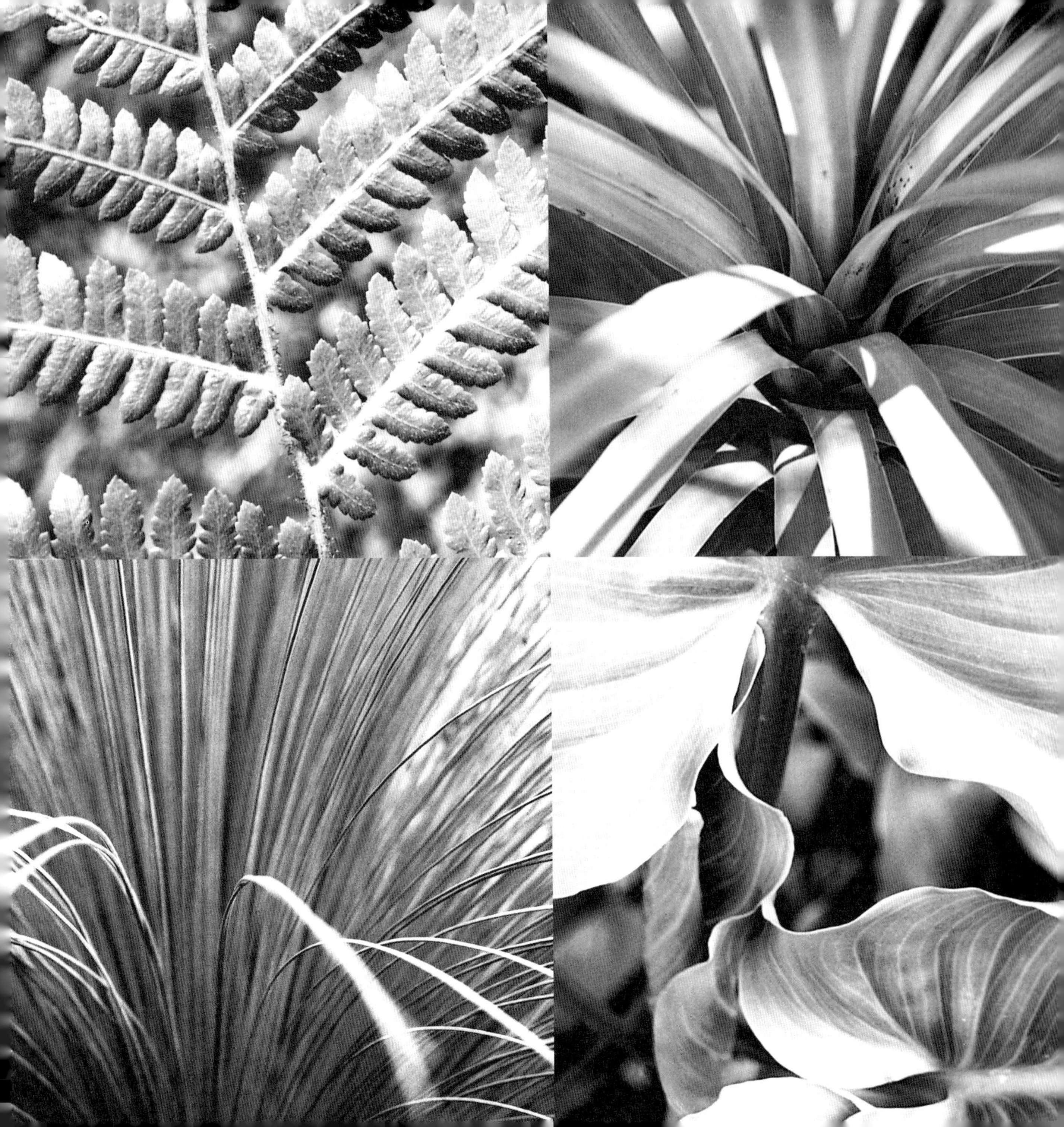

Sacred Wood

There are symbols and events from cultures and traditions around the world that we can use to speak about the qualities of the Chinese Wood element.

The Bodhi tree is a symbol of wisdom, attainment, enlightenment and the potential of humans to transcend worldly existence. In India some 2500 years ago, the meditating Shakyamuni Buddha achieved enlightenment under the Bodhi tree, a type of fig. People still visit the site at Bodh Gaya where the original tree stood. The Buddha triumphed over illusion and became the living embodiment of wisdom and compassion.

The olive branch symbolises the ideal of peace on earth and our continuing quest for this peace. When we 'hold out the olive branch' we gesture that we are interested in tolerance and understanding. In the biblical story of the ark a dove brought an olive branch to Noah as a symbol that life on Earth could peacefully resume after the turbulent floods. Many flags, including that of the United Nations, use the olive branch as a symbol of unity. The olive tree itself is often regarded as 'the tree of life', particularly in the Middle East.

The Ancient Grecian forest God, Pan, is nature personified in a body that is half man and half goat. Pan plays the flute, the purest of the wind instruments; wind is the traditional 'climate' associated with the Wood element (see page 169). Pan can cause people to become enraged with anger, which is the emotional challenge of the traditional Chinese Wood element. When Pan's influence becomes too strong people may panic and lose control. Control is an attribute of the Wood element.

The spring (Vernal) equinox brings a celebration of new beginnings, resurrection and the commencement of life; spring is the season of Wood energy. Equinox winds may roam the land and bring a sense of clearance and change. When the sun is in the sky for exactly twelve hours, rises exactly in the East, sets exactly in the West, we experience the order and equilibrium that typifies the energy of the Wood element.

Windows of the soul

The liver, which is the Yin organ of the Wood element, houses the soul (*hun* in Chinese). Traditional Chinese Medicine doesn't consider the soul to be separate from the living person in the same way that many other cultures do. Healing practices based on Traditional Chinese Medicine don't address a person's body without considering the emotions, the spirit and the soul. In many ways it is the soul that is first addressed; the health of the soul is seen as imperative to overall well-being.

The eyes are the sense organs of Wood energy; they relate in particular to the *liver* channel. Imagine an energetic interconnecting system that links the associations and functions of the elements within our bodies along a series of channels. In this case the association is the eyes, which are primarily governed by the Wood element's *liver* channel. Although Wood energy is concerned with liver function and opens into the eyes, the network can't be segmented for discussion in Traditional Chinese Medicine because the interactions are so intertwined. To say that poor eyesight is the result of liver problems is only a brushstroke on a very large canvas — every person is unique.

There is a saying that 'the eyes are the windows of the soul'. People everywhere, consciously or unconsciously, gauge from these sense organs the innermost nature of a person. Eyes are the softest tissue material that we expose to the external world and are the only part of our bodies we withdraw in the vulnerability of sleep. They are our primary connection to the daylight world and represent the 'driver's seat' for the vehicle of our body. They feed our brain with the images of our surroundings; they are the mediators of primary exchange. When we become depressed or lose the sense of new beginnings that the Wood element brings to us we withdraw from life and our eyes may weaken, particularly after emotional crisis. A great weariness and sadness can be seen in the eyes of those who carry burdens, as can a great sparkling light from the eyes of those who have found contentment in life and continue to be excited by the possibilities of things to come.

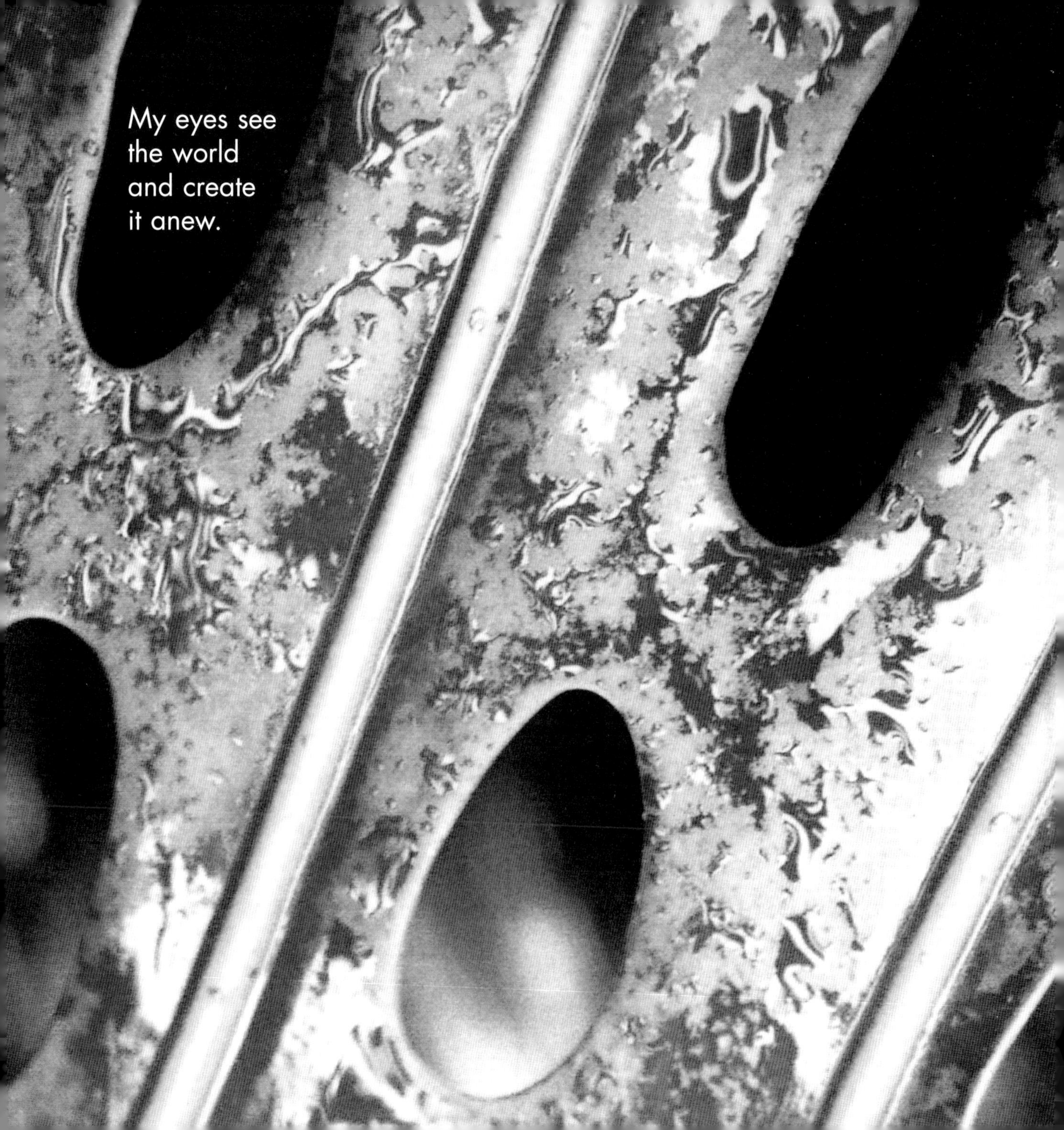
My eyes see
the world
and create
it anew.

Meditation on Wood

Let your body and mind come to be present in this moment and place. Sit comfortably in your meditation posture — relaxed yet upright, alert and aware.

Have your eyes softly open, focused on the ground just ahead of you. Your lips are lightly closed and your tongue rests against the top palate of your mouth.

Bring your attention to your breathing.

Watch your breath as it moves in and out of your body. Allow a visualisation to gently guide you: as you breathe in and feel the expansion of your belly, have the awareness of a seed resting deep in your belly.

Focus your attention on this 'seed' for a few minutes while you continue to breathe.

Now, with the in-breath, begin to fill your body with a beautiful light, the colour of forest green. Let it start at your feet and flood up through your body, up through your trunk and limbs until it reaches the crown of your head and fills you entirely. This green is cleansing and invigorating and makes you feel strong. It is vibrant with life force, yet remains calm. It fills you with inspiration and optimism and brings new vision to your life.

Now bring your attention to your out-breath. The sound of your out-breath is like a thousand leaves whispering in the wind: it is a sigh that releases the tensions and restraints within your body and soul, leaving you supple and soft like a frond in the beginnings of new growth.

Continue breathing in the cleansing light of green and breathing out all the old patterns of your life — the 'dead wood' of your past.

This is a new beginning, a regrowth.

This is a time of spring cleansing.

Stay with these images for a time until your breathing is purposeful and ordered, with an easy, organic rhythm.

When your meditation nears an end, gradually slow the movement of your breath, and of your visualisation, until the breath is so gentle it is almost imperceptible — the softest breeze.

Let your mind find a quiet place deep in a beautiful lush green forest, and rest there.

During the day contemplate the words 'flexibility' and 'harmony'.

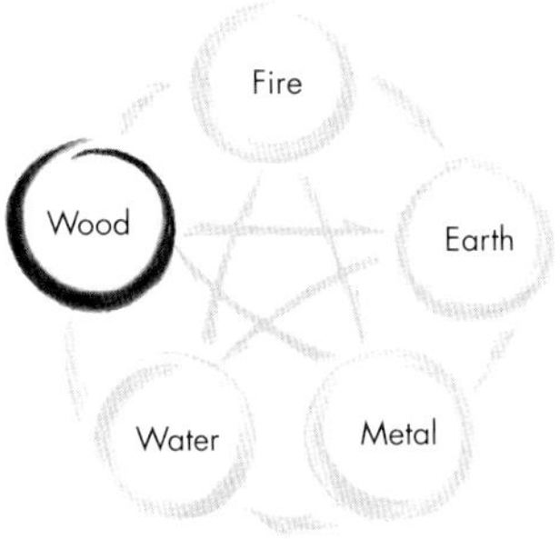

Wood energy in Traditional Chinese Medicine

The General of the Army

I am the General in charge of all the armies of the realm. My will is to impose order, my destiny is to control and protect. I am driven, decisive and ambitious and I have the qualities of a great leader. Whether I attract followers is another matter. That depends on how well I administer my virtue of flexibility when I plan, organise and act!

The Wood element channels and important points

The Yin and Yang channels of my Wood element are called *liver* and *gall bladder*. They take these names from the organs in which Wood Qi activity is most evident. As my *liver* and *gall bladder* energy channels flow up and down my body they cover a wide area, which they supply with Qi. When I have any problems with pain, the liver Qi is always involved because part of its function is to dredge the channels of 'stuck Qi'.

- Pain always means there is blockage of normal Qi flow. I will need the spreading attributes of the third point of the *liver* channel, *Taichong*, meaning 'Great Thoroughfare'.
- When I am depressed or despairing and my faith in life is diminished I choose 'Gate of Hope', *Qimen*, the fourteenth point on the *liver* channel, to help me release the past and open my eyes to a new day.
- When I am vanquished and my Wood energy spent, or when I am elderly, I need the first point on the *liver* channel, *Dadun*, meaning 'Great Sincerity'. It is the Wood point on this Wood channel and will bring me substance and sustenance.

The Wood element within our body, mind and emotions

Body

The liver and gall bladder are the companion organs of my Wood element. The *liver* channel controls my eyes, muscles and tendons, and nourishes my blood. It stores my blood at night and if upset cannot hold it correctly. This will disrupt my sleep and my ability to properly nourish the muscles and eyes, leading to weakness.

Emotional problems block the flow of my *liver* Qi. Unresolved conflicts, denial and stress all hinder my desire for swift and decisive movement. This causes stagnation and dams the flow of Qi causing it to turn to heat and burn my Wood. Heat causes my Qi to rise and it will often gather at the neck and shoulders, causing chronic tightness. Eventually the dam bursts and a large amount of fiery *liver* energy is released suddenly upwards, which can cause headaches; or it may strike sideways and cause gastric upsets.

Wood element channels in the body

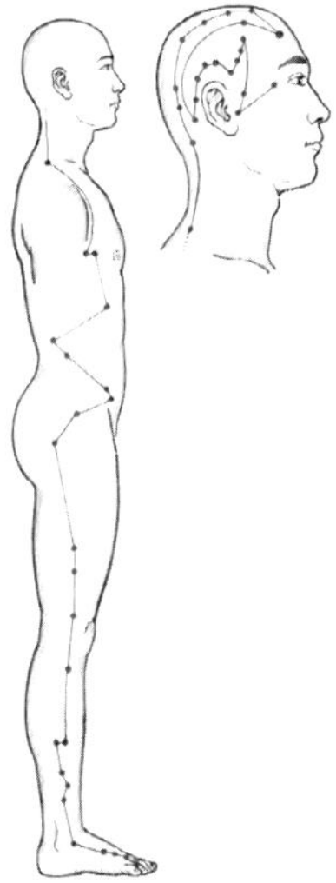

Gall Bladder — Yang channel of Wood

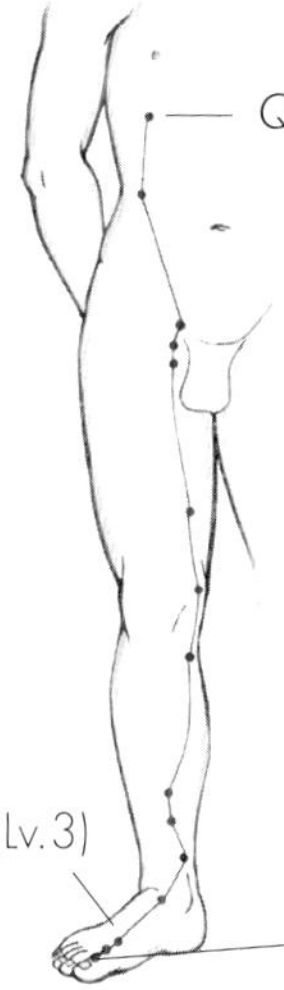

Liver — Yin channel of Wood

When my Wood constitution is unbalanced I can appear abrasive and defensive, indecisive or 'stuck'. I am clever at maintaining control of my appearance and I will often wear a face over my anger. This causes further blockages and more problems. My remedy often involves nourishing and harmonising my Wood element and clearing stagnation from the energy channels. Exercise, expressing emotions and learning to bend with the breeze are often simple remedies to which I respond well.

Mind

Vision and strategic thinking are the natural talents of my Wood element. When I project these qualities in a positive way, order can be assured. If I am overzealous or too controlling, tyranny and rebellion can reign in my physical, mental and emotional worlds. A disruption to any part of the process from thought to action can result in stagnation, which is distressing to my element. Movement is all-important to the nature of my Wood energy.

Emotions

I can be inflexible, intolerant and prone to fiery outbursts as my Wood element energy burns for release. Anger is my principle emotion; yet my Wood phase is also responsible for processing and harmonising all of the emotions — including anger.

If I become paralysed with fear, my anger can be used to keep me stuck, making me stubborn and shortsighted; yet anger can also give me the courage to break free from my limitations. Previously unseen pathways are opened by anger, and my vision is sharpened. Properly expressed, anger is a valued companion to harmonious order. Tears are associated with *liver* Qi; they soften the sometimes brittle nature of my Wood element, allowing me the optimism of new growth.

Destiny of the Wood element

With careful organisation, I harness an irrepressible passion for life. The spirit of my Wood element projects a destiny of tolerance, benevolent protection and ease.

Humility tempers my healthy yet boisterous Wood nature. I am quick to initiate ideas and I know how to get support from those around me. I respond to change with flexibility and adjust quickly to changes outside my control.

The tree bending
in the wind survives
the storm.

The supple does
not break, the
flexible endures.

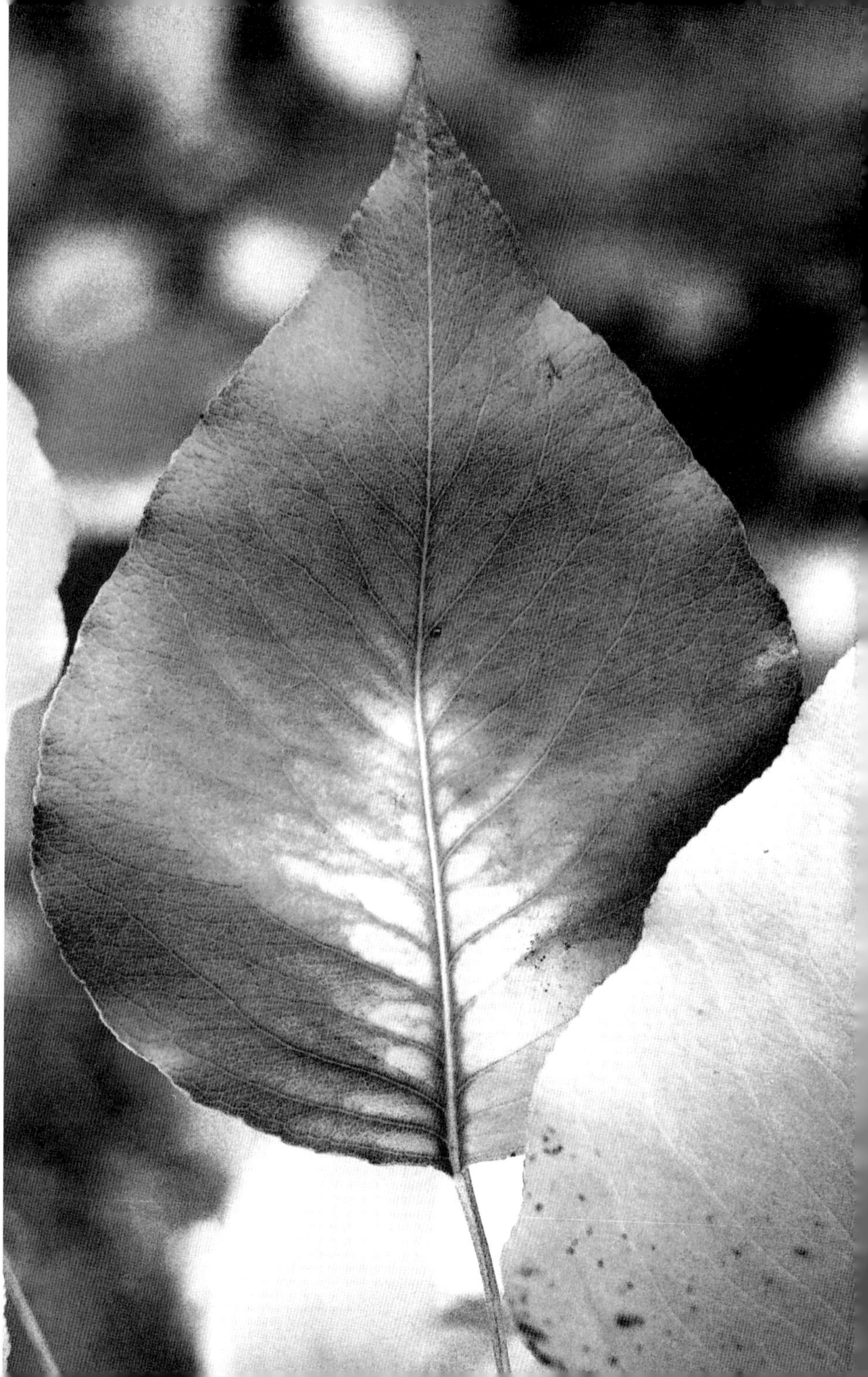

Fire

I dance in the passionate heat of summer,
joy fills my heart.
My brilliant light glows in hues of vibrant red,
my flames give warmth, and gather you close to me.
I am enthusiastic and alive!
The source of elation.

I house the Shen, the spirit of your being.
I am sacred, pure and sensitive,
protected and protective.
I lose heart if neglected,
and can be broken by the careless
or the emotionally barren.

I am the sun, laughing and listening —
respect my power!
Unchecked, I scorch and consume,
harnessed I bear ripeness and fruition.

I am dynamic, and my will is done.
I am art, music and language,
pulsating with life blood, and desire.
I am creation and destruction,
vital, devastatingly beautiful —
the spark of all life.

I am the energy of Fire.

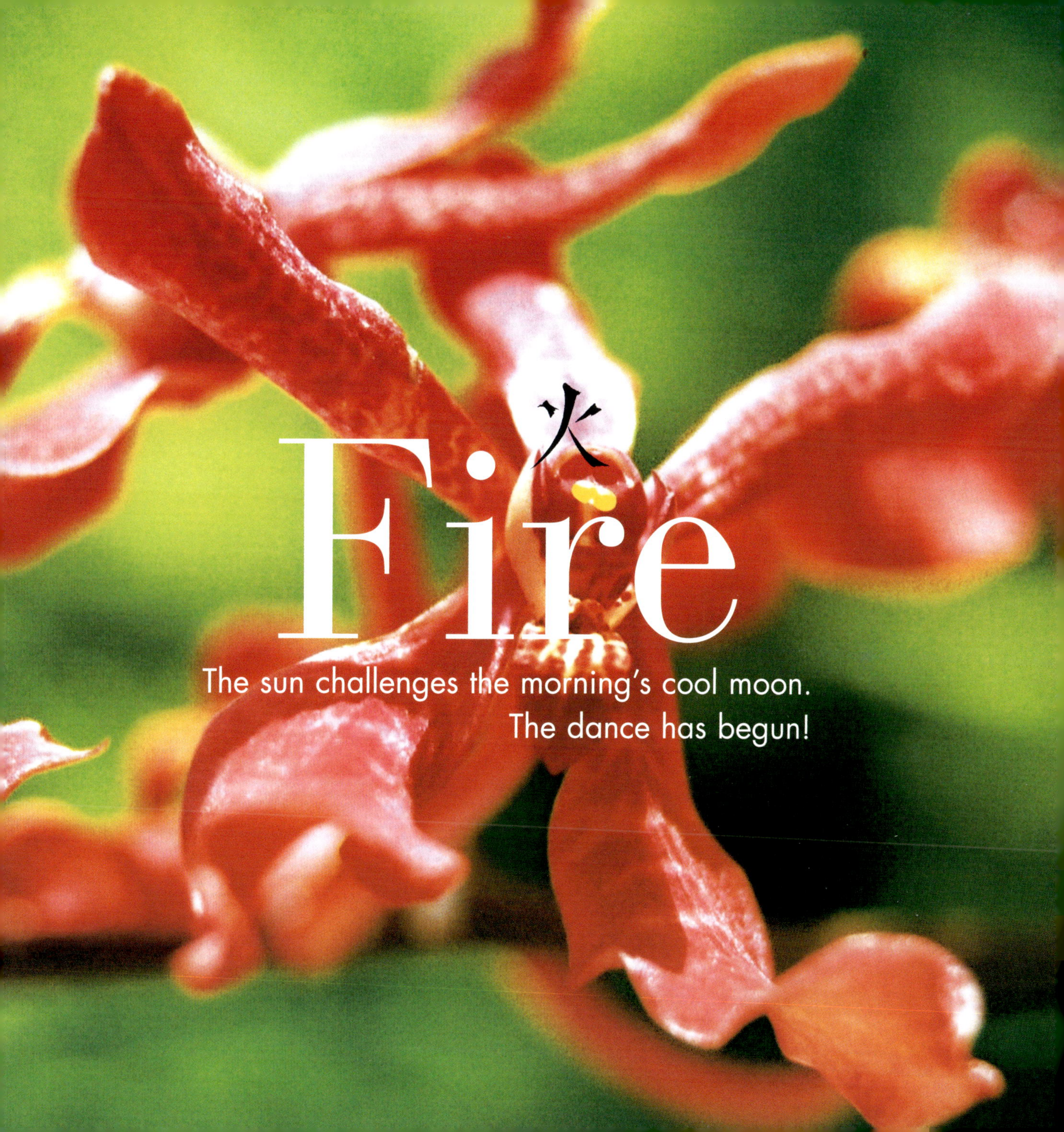

火 Fire

The sun challenges the morning's cool moon.
The dance has begun!

Traditional Chinese Fire element associations:

Summer, red, joy, laughing, the tongue, blood and vessels, the small intestine, the heart, the pericardium, the three burners, the south, heat, the bitter tastes.

The Fire element expressed in nature

At the pinnacle of the five phases is an explosion of colour and light. Fire energy bursts into life, dancing languidly with a passionate joy. In Five Element theory the direction or essential movement of fire is outward in all directions from the centre — the flames reach out in a fearless, optimistic search.

The brilliance of fire substance draws beings to its warmth; fire is the essential warmth existing in all earthly life. The dynamic spark that begins life is seen in the creation of the earth itself: new land is born with an explosive expression of fire from deep within the heart of the planet, which cools to shape our mountains and fertile volcanic plains. In Chinese Five Element theory the Fire element is the traditional creator of the Earth element in the Sheng construction cycle.

Fire substance will burn what fuel is given and can be a joy to watch. But the same fire that warms our blood grows suddenly frightening when it has too much wood, because the Wood element is the creator of the Fire element in the Sheng cycle. Fire can flood through space and devour everything in its path with a relentless enthusiasm, until it is exhausted again; until everything is 'burnt out' in the excitement, in the heat of the moment.

This destruction always begins a cycle of creation. Fire can be the energy that triggers regeneration and continuation. For ecosystems such as Australian eucalypt forests, fire is part of the natural order: the seeds are activated by the heat and smoke, and the trees sprout new green shoots. The open tree canopy allows light to reach the forest floor, which is covered in ash and nutrients to nourish the seedlings.

We cannot make wood, water, rock or earth in the way that we can make fire. Through alchemy we transform the manifestations of the elements, but the energy of fire is readily available. It is a vital ingredient in many acts of alchemy, both ancient and new.

Fire,
the creator,
celebrates life
and love,
and is sensitive
to changes
in nature.

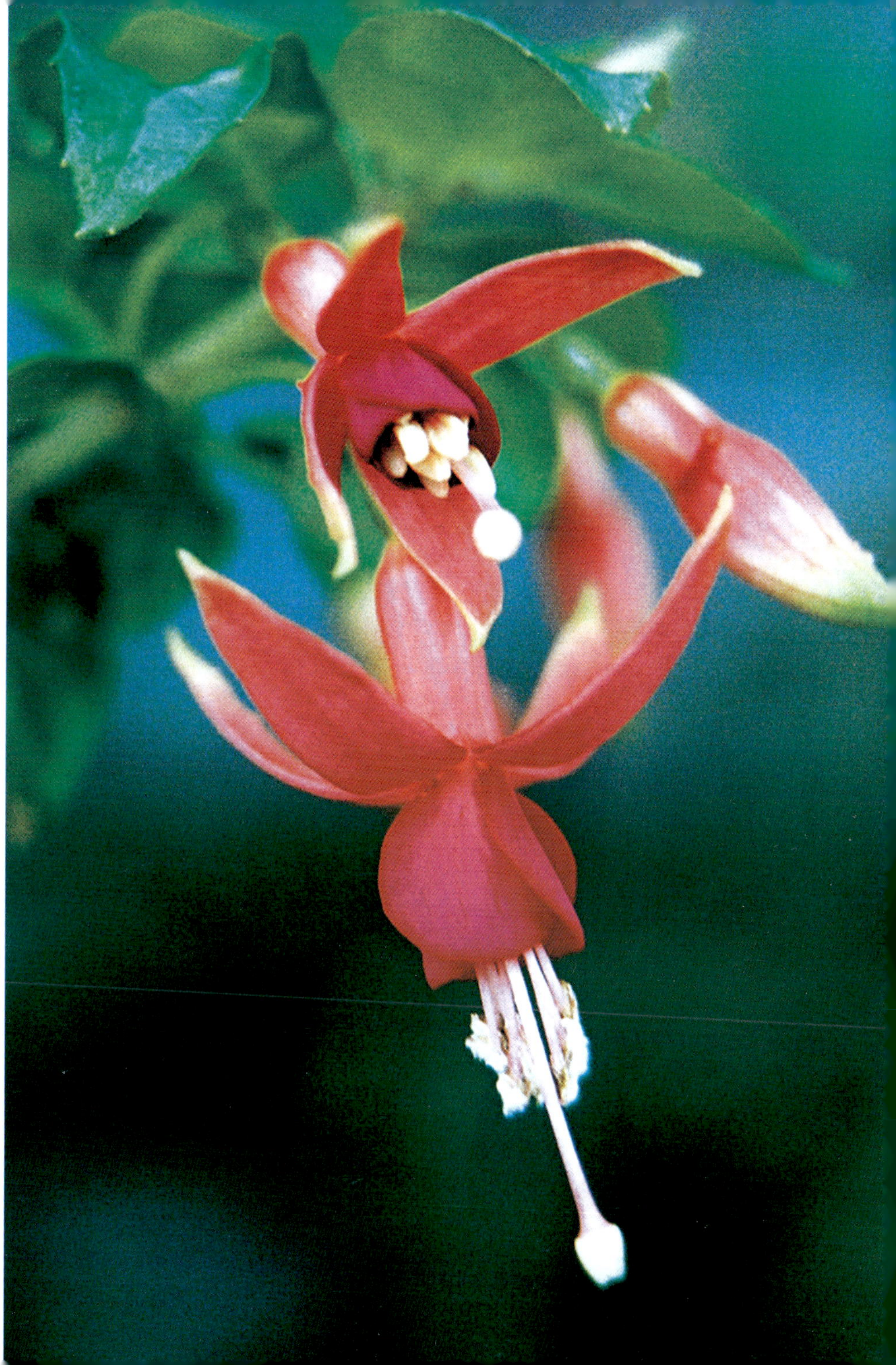

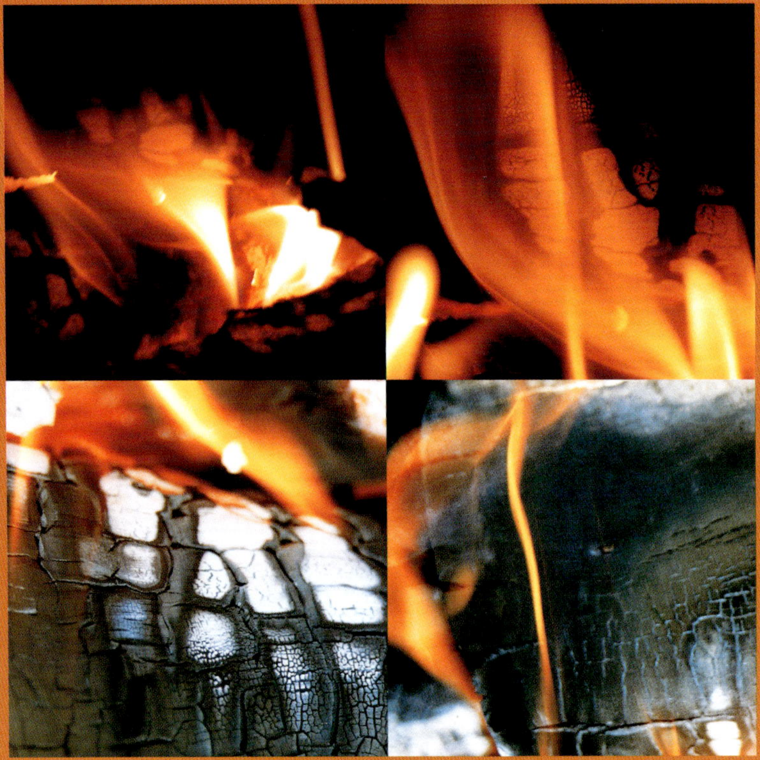

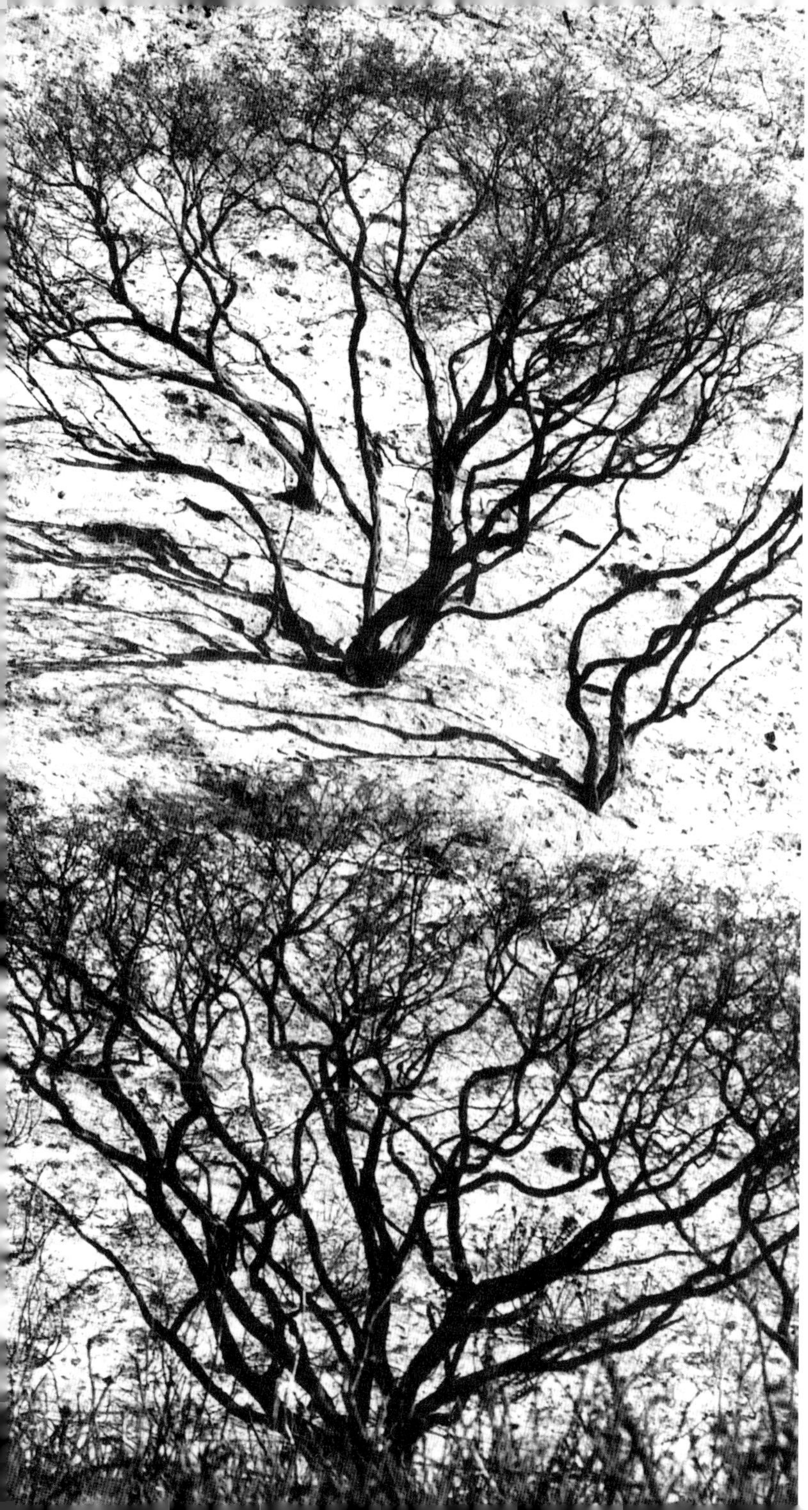

The Fire element is the supreme 'emperor' of the Five Element cycle. Everything fire touches in nature is changed. Water is transformed to steam — disembodied; wood loses substance and becomes ash; earth is baked hard or created from volcanic activity — as is Metal (rock and stone), which in turn can be melted into liquid.

Fire is very much a living element in nature. When a fire sparks into life, we understand that it is transient and will enjoy a limited life; the fire is constantly rekindling, subsiding, and starting again afresh. It can be in a million different places at once, wherever the opportunity and conditions exist. The Fire element bestows us with the joy of a transient dance on earth.

Fire and the house of Shen

The consciousness of our nature — of our spirit — is housed within the Fire element of our being and is called 'Shen'. Sometimes Shen is understood to mean the spirit of an individual, but in the Chinese Five Element system our spirit is not an entity apart. The idea of housing the Shen is all-important. The Fire element plays a protective role in the body, and in Traditional Chinese Medicine the pericardium — the minder and guardian of the heart — falls under Fire's control.

When we watch flames dancing in a hearth our thoughts are free to transcend the mundane world: Fire energy brings us visions and divine guidance. The presence of the Fire element brings focus to our Shen — our spiritual self — and encourages us to explore spontaneous imagery and elevating ideas. Wherever there is fire, people will gather to tell stories, sing songs or share their innermost thoughts and aspirations. Children especially love the experience of a camp fire or bonfire.

The Fire element offers the excitement of possibility and enriches the visions of the artist, the poet and the prophet. Fire energy sates our passion for vision and spirited expression.

The Fire element brings illumination to our being. The Shen lights the way to acts of spiritual creativity; the dark shuns this light and is dispelled. Fire illuminates a path with the brilliance of its nature. We move on this path with a feeling of joy in our hearts — the emotional gift of the Fire element. We understand that fire demands spontaneous acceptance of this gift, of this happiness.

Fire is the house of divine affection and the active nature of creation.

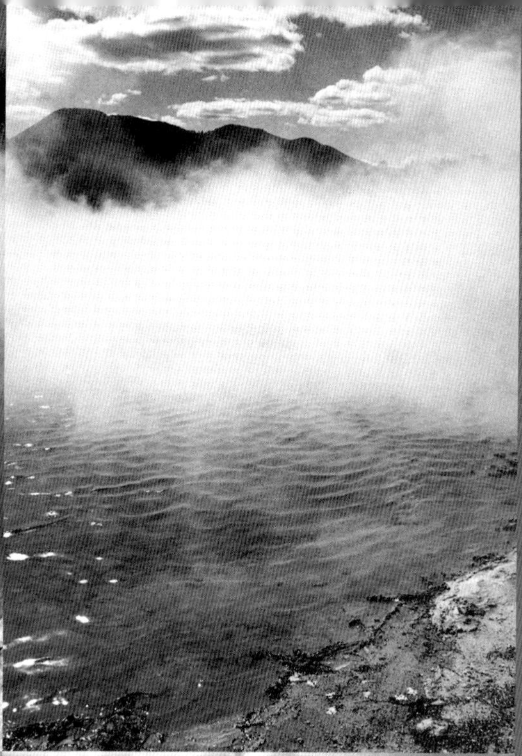

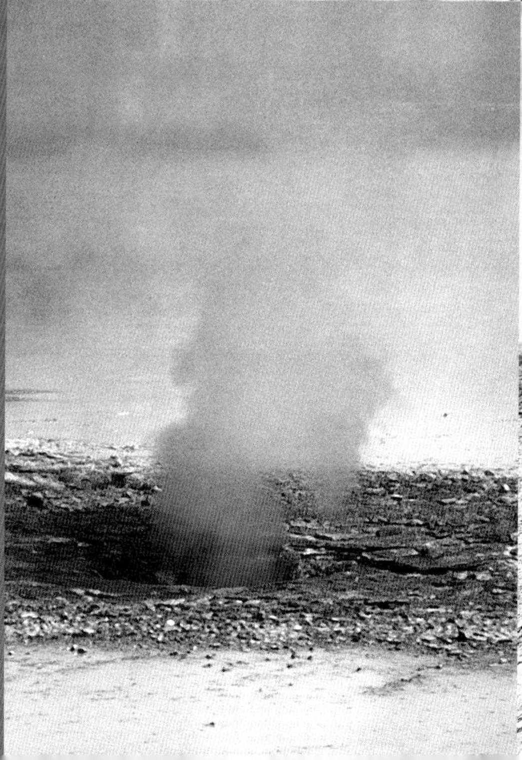

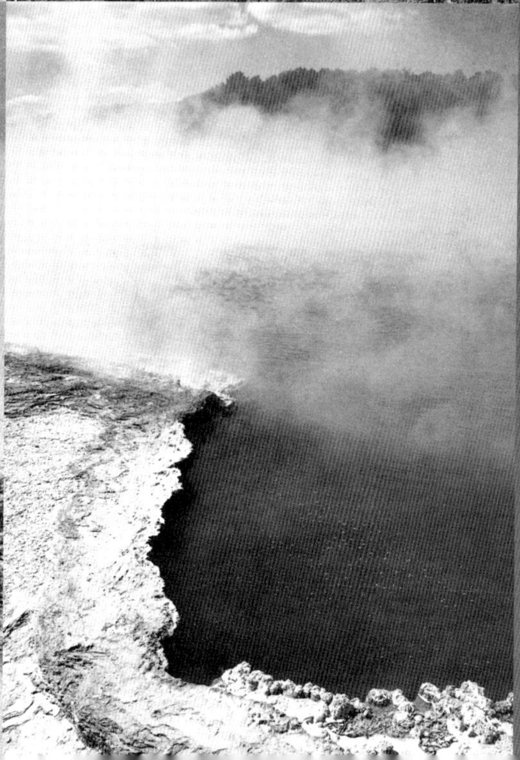

Sacred Fire

In Greek and some Polynesian mythologies people share versions of a story in which fire once belonged to the gods. Humans stole or received fire as a gift from these gods (such as Prometheus) and are now the caretakers of its creative power.

Whatever icons we use for revering fire, it is the Fire element within our bodies — living in our hearts — that we must protect most strongly. The energetic influence of the Fire element brings to our lives creativity, passion, joy and a love of magic.

There are symbolic practices and natural phenomena from around the world that illustrate the qualities of the Fire element.

The sun, our daytime star, is perhaps the ultimate iconic manifestation of the Fire element in action. This enormous body of broiling fire bestows the warmth and light by which we live, and by which our planet maintains a predetermined course through the solar system. The sun literally illuminates our lives as we spin through the blackness of space; it takes the role of supreme control over the elements. (In traditional Five Element theory, Fire is the 'Emperor' of the Five Elements.)

Fireworks are sometimes used as a ritual tool for the occult purpose of driving away negative or malefic entities, especially in beginning a new year. They symbolise transcendence of our earthly concerns and the purifying force of the Fire element.

Lightning often symbolises divine power or the source of original fire.

The eternal flame burns in sacred honour of ideals and higher beings, or in remembrance of the spirits of those departed.

A funeral pyre is seen as a purification of the soul and the liberator of the spirit, a severance from the material world. When our bodies are committed to fire all but a handful of ashes is consumed without trace and is returned to the soil and air. Our spirit is freed.

A candle can be used to symbolically represent communion with God, the higher self, or the spiritual realm. As the Fire element is the house of the spirit, the candle flame is symbolic of spiritual illumination. Candles may be lit as an act of atonement, or purely as a symbol of reverence for things divine.

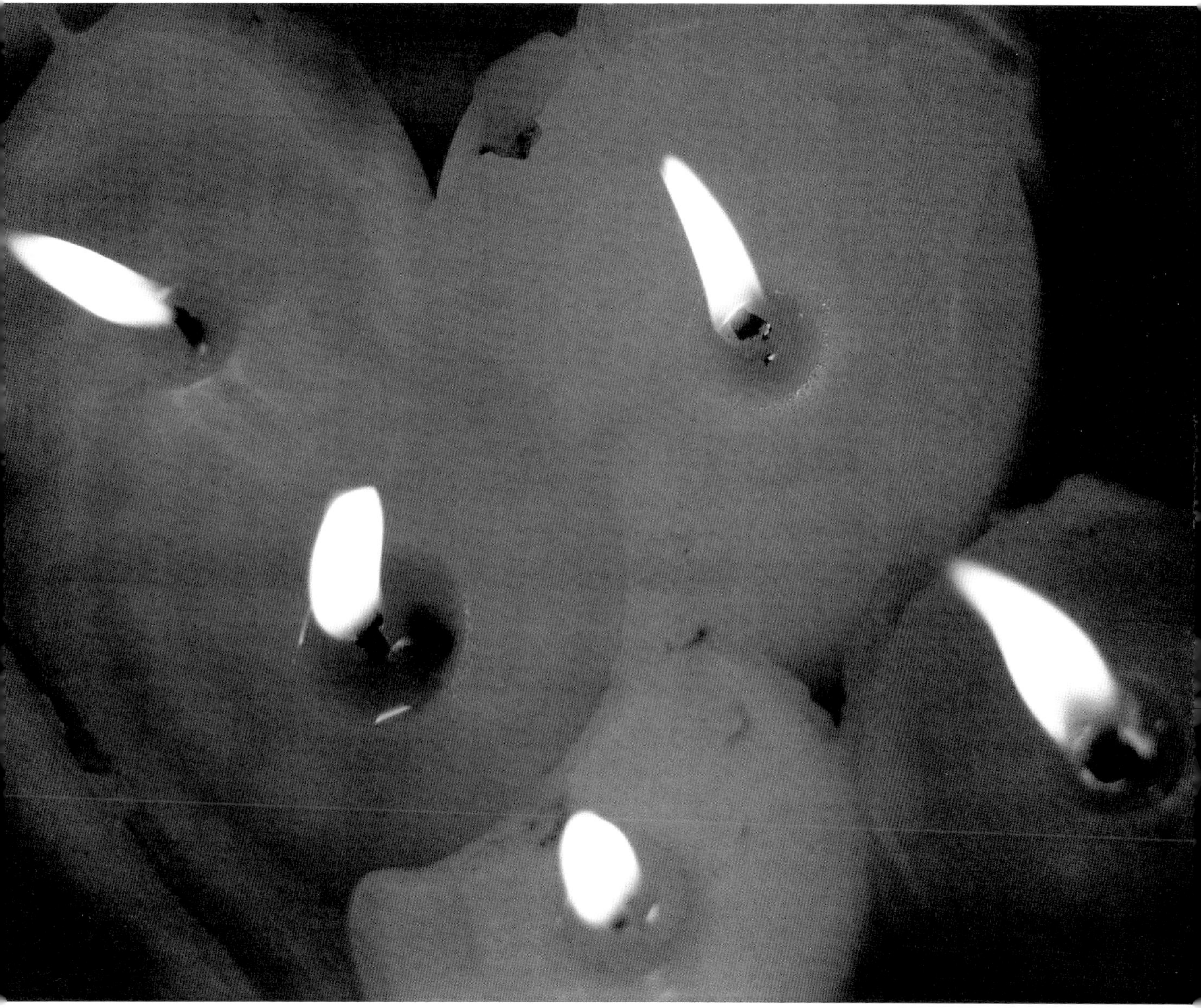

Passions

The Fire element ignites in us a passion to move and to dance. In summer, the season of fire, blood surges through our body, warmed by the sun. We laugh aloud as the brilliant light banishes the dark of winter; all things ripen to be enjoyed at this succulent peak of existence. Fire is life — the very pulse of our being.

In Five Element theory, Fire associates closely with the heart, which is also the home of romantic emotional attachment in most cultures. Any heart-felt emotion is one that is deeply moving and that touches the very heart of our beings, the consciousness of our spiritual self.

To have a fire in your belly is to be driven, to be 'fired up' and 'inflamed'. When the creative juices are flowing we feel excitement for life and a sense of heightened awareness. Artists will paint into the night, musicians will play their instruments with a transcendent vigour, and the muse will drive the hands of the sculptor.

Red is the colour of our life-blood and the traditional colour of the Fire element. We associate red with love, passion, sex and desire. When the Fire element is strong within us we can allow our thoughts to wander freely between the world of desire, the realm of spirit, and the active world of primary creative expression. Fire dares us to live a life of passion.

Passion reaches for a place beyond time.

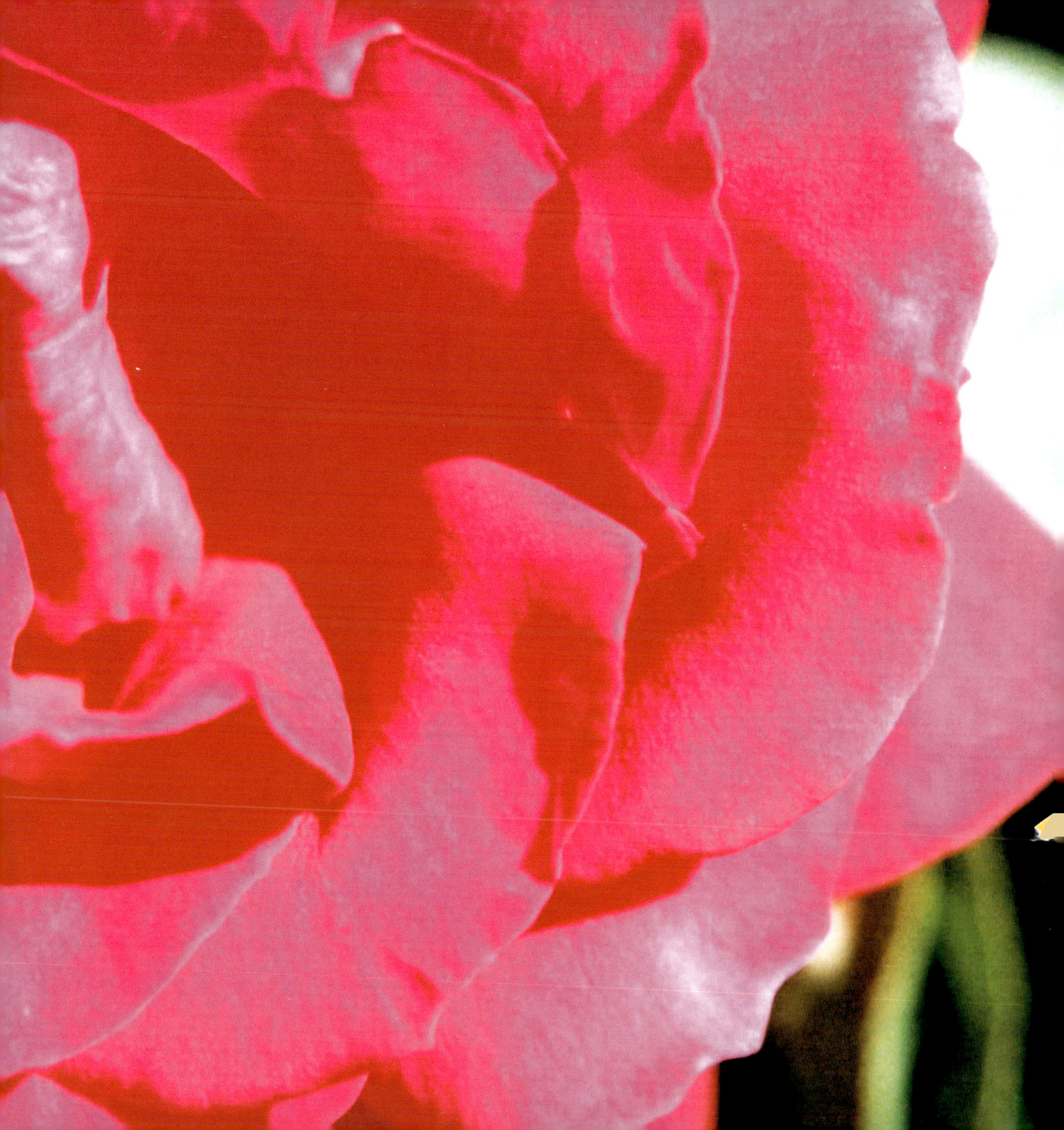

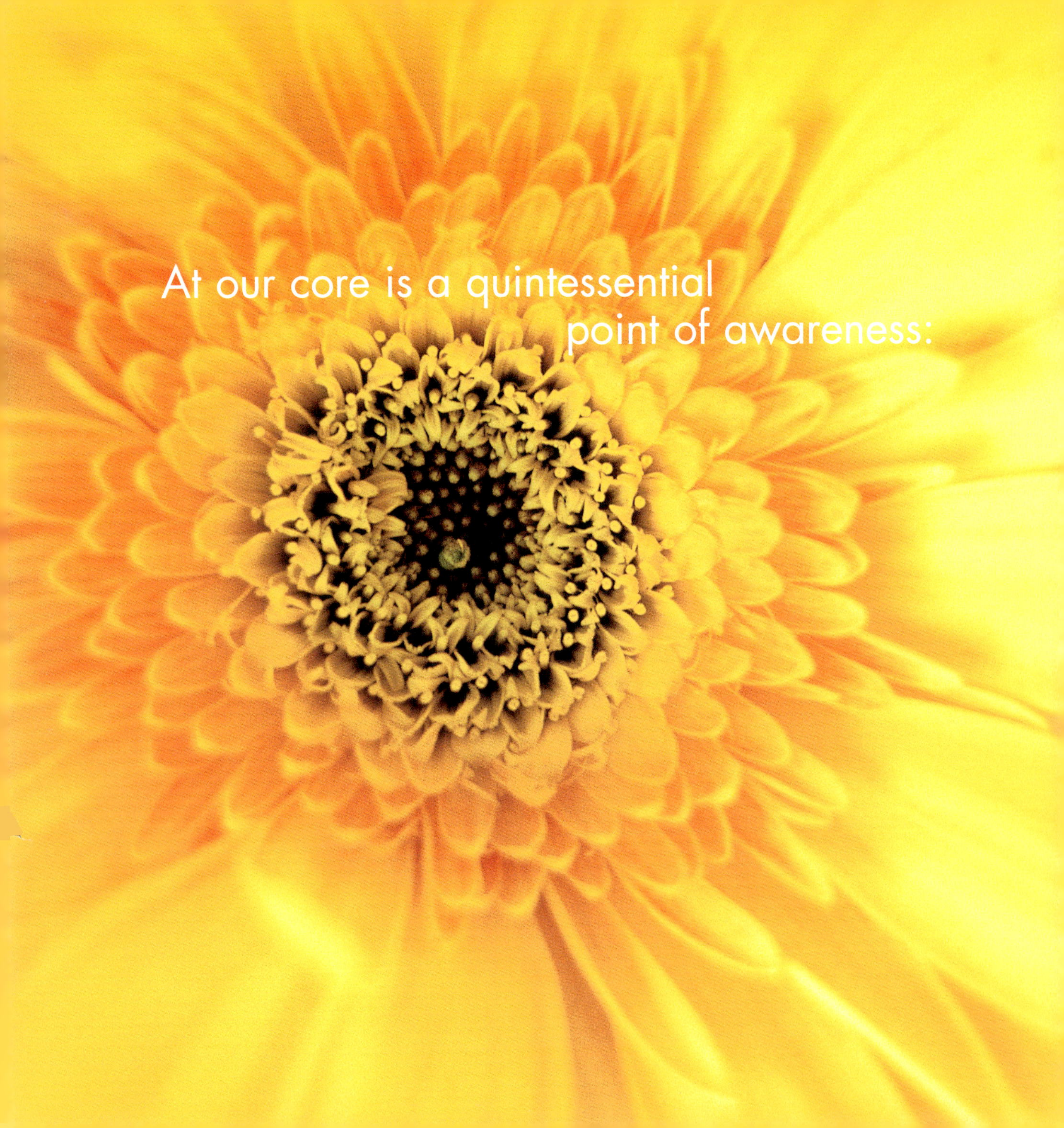
At our core is a quintessential
point of awareness:

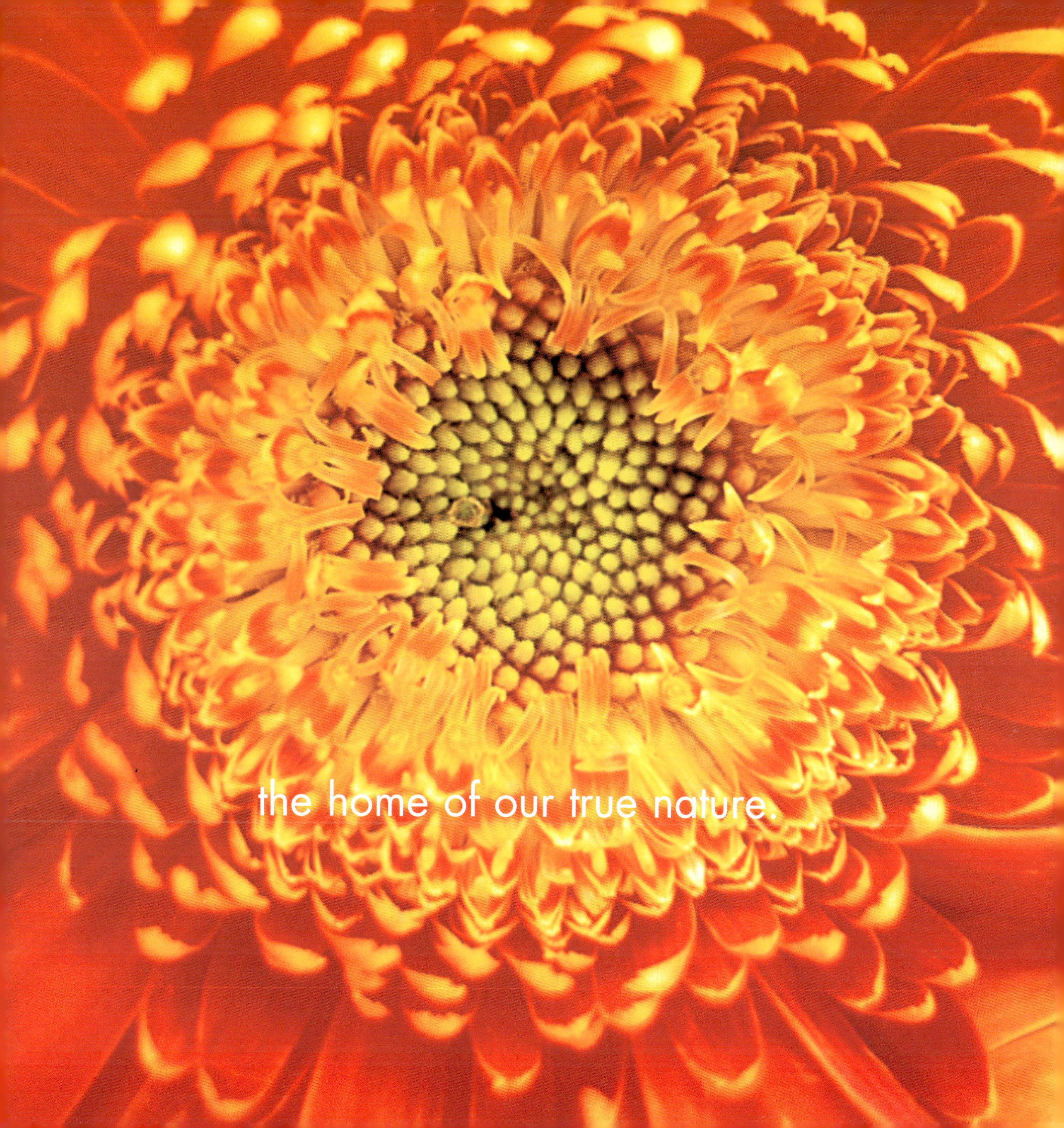
the home of our true nature.

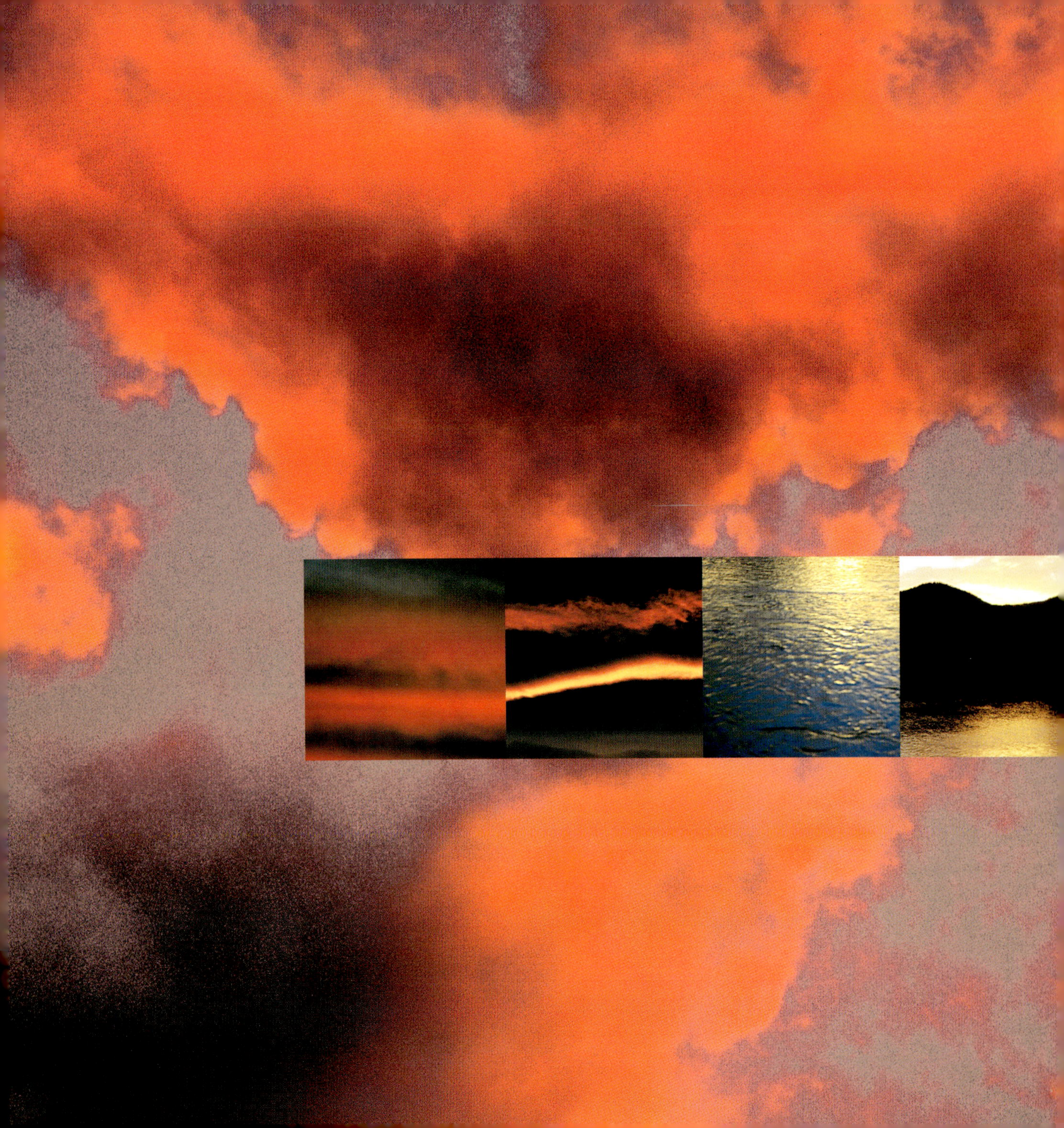

Laughter

In Five Element theory, Fire affords us the capacity for speech. The way in which we speak can reflect dispositions or tendencies concerned with any of the elements, but the ability to speak and the nature of speech is concerned with the tongue and with Fire. Verbal communication is an important creative tool for the active expression of fire within our bodies, as is laughter, which is the sound traditionally attributed to Fire energy. When we hear someone laugh it is easy to visualise a fire flaring up and dancing on the spot. It is contagious and lifts our spirits. Like a fire, it jumps from place to place.

Disciplines and practices that move towards achieving enlightenment often use the absence of speech over long periods of time as a tool for diminishing attachment to worldly phenomena. How interesting that these same people often carry great laughter and joy in their eyes!

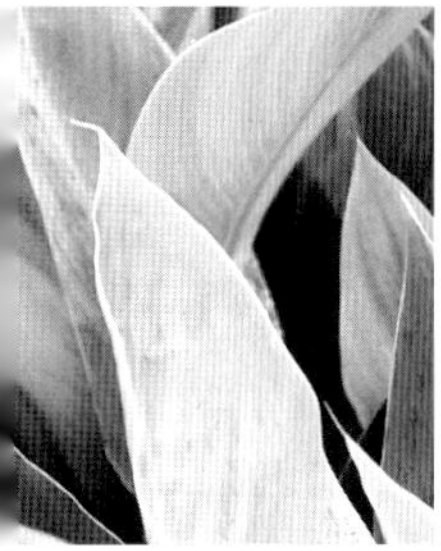

Fire lights a way in the dark and laughs at the shadows.

When we laugh we feel released from our fears and sorrows and enjoy the pure elation of being alive. The shadows are banished as our joy shines a light on the world, and we begin to heal old wounds and to cleanse our spirit. Laughter is often 'the best medicine'.

Action!

At the top of a flame the energy of fire focuses its intentions like a point on a dagger or the tip of a Japanese sumi-e ink brush. The Fire element is the outward (extroverted) expression of the inward (introverted) workings — the spearhead of the 'elemental spear'.

Fire is the Element of action and the representation of activity in its most dynamically embodied form. In a theatre production the actor in the spotlight can be likened to the tip of the flame; this person is likely to have strong Fire element influences. Those backstage — scenery-makers, props people, wardrobe and make-up, crew and technicians — are likely to have other elements as their strong influences.

Fire is sensitive to its surroundings and needs support, encouragement and even some fans! But when Fire energy does come to life it is dynamic and powerful and glows with a light of its own.

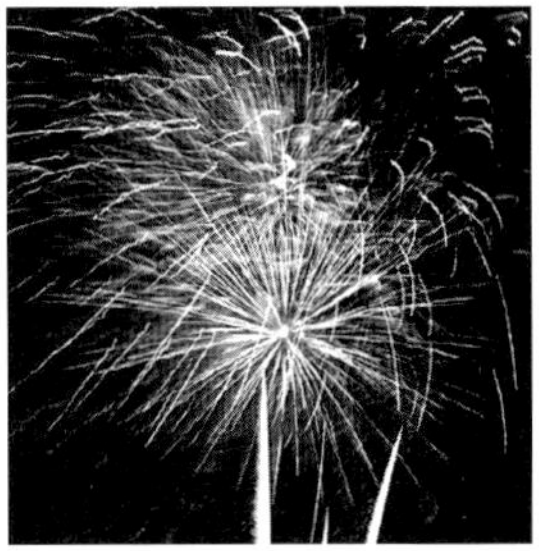

Elation is the animating essence that fuels our spirited Fire.

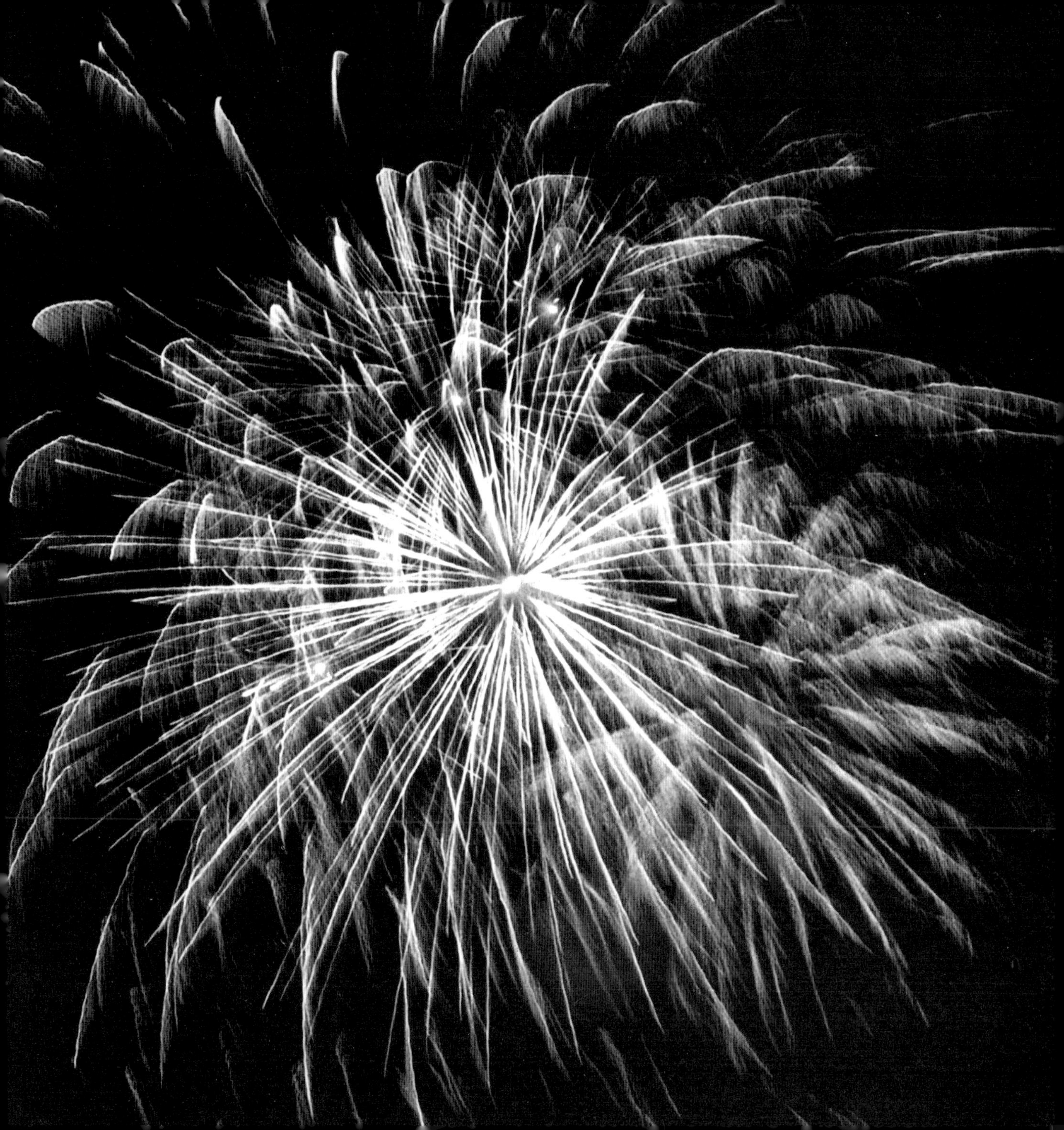

Meditation on Fire

Let your body and mind come to be present in this moment and place. Sit comfortably in your meditation posture before a lit fireplace or a candle, your eyes gently focused on the flame. Your lips are lightly closed, and your tongue rests against the top palate of your mouth.

Bring your attention to your breathing and smile into your belly. Watch your breath as it moves in and out of your body. It is strong and rhythmic.

With one hand, squeeze the tip of the small finger on the other — just below the nail on either side of the finger. Parallel with the cuticle you'll find an indent that is sensitive. These are Fire points.

Bring your joined hands to your belly, just above your navel on your solar plexus. This will create warmth in your body. (You can use a pillow or 'belt' made from your meditation shawl to support your hands.)

Your breath comes in through your nose and greets the feeling of warmth beginning to form in your belly. Allow this in-breath to surround itself around the warmth, and to create an imaginary sphere of crackling embers, to stimulate the fire within.

The out-breath comes through the mouth — your lips now form a gentle 'O' shape — and the sound is like a bellows being blown onto embers. The fire flares and storms through the body, calming as the out-breath ends. This is the ultimate cleansing and brings joy to your heart.

Again the in-breath surrounds and excites the embers in your belly. Again the out-breath frees the fire and causes it to whoosh around the body until its fuel of air is exhausted.

As the fire grows in your body, you may begin to breathe out some of the flame, like a dragon, but keep plenty of warmth for yourself.

After a time, quieten your breath, release your hand, and sit quietly with your eyes softly focused on the candle flame.

The energy of Fire remains in your body and the glow will bring warmth to those around you.

During the day contemplate the joy of gratitude.

Note to meditation

If you have high blood pressure or a heart condition, you may wish to blow out all of the fire on the out-breath, or choose another element for your meditation. If you begin to feel very hot in the face stop the meditation and splash your head and face with some cool water.

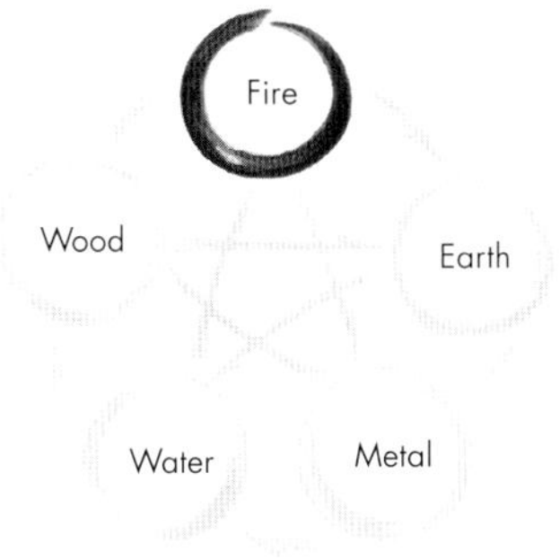

Fire energy in Traditional Chinese Medicine

The Emperor

I am the Emperor in supreme control of all the elements! I bring peace, as my destiny is to inspire harmony between heaven and earth. I radiate light and joy as I am in communion with the divine. Omnipotent and wise, I exercise fair judgement in sorting the pure from the impure and the material from the immaterial. How well I listen to my heart centre will determine the depth and quality of my worldly relationships.

The Fire element channels and important points

The four channels of the Fire element all begin or end on the fingers. The two Yang channels of this element reach the head and the two Yin channels issue forth from my thorax. The channels take their names from the two organs that most closely associate with the Fire element — *heart* and *small intestine* — and from two observed Qi functions in the body that do not include physical organs — *three burners* and *pericardium*. Fire is the only element that has four basic channels attributed to it.

- When I am feeling sad and shut off from life I choose heart point number three, *Shaohai*, meaning 'Lesser Sea'. This can help to encourage a state of *joie de vivre*.
- If I am suffering palpitations or an irregular heartbeat I can use *Neiguan*, meaning 'Inner Gate', to harmonise and balance Fire. This is the sixth point on the *pericardium* channel.

- If my dreams are upsetting or if I am restless and agitated, *heart* point seven, *Shenmen*, 'Spirit Gate', will free me to calmly reconnect with my spirit. I will feel content.
- Exhaustion and serious heart illness may require *heart* point number one, *Shaochong*, or 'Lesser Rushing', the Wood point on the *heart* channel. This point nourishes the heart through the Mother–Child relationship, where Wood is the mother of Fire.

Fire element channels in the body

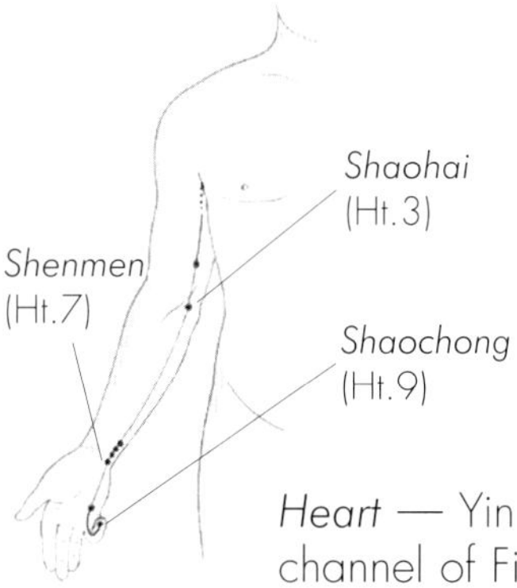

Heart — Yin channel of Fire

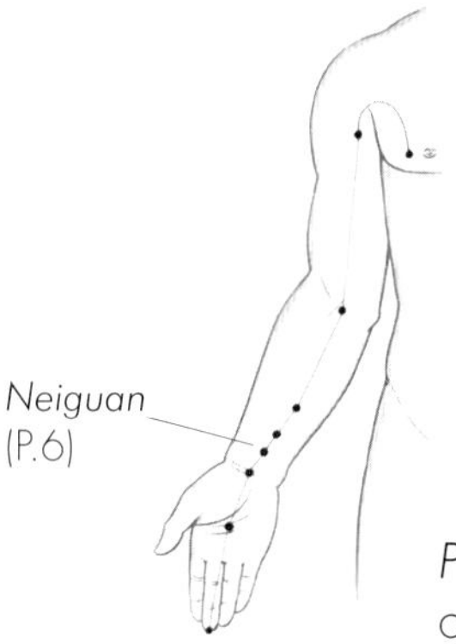

Pericardium — Yin channel of Fire

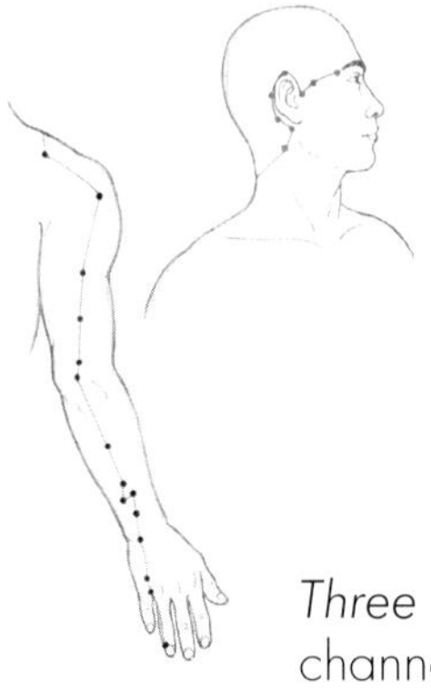

Three Burners — Yang channel of Fire

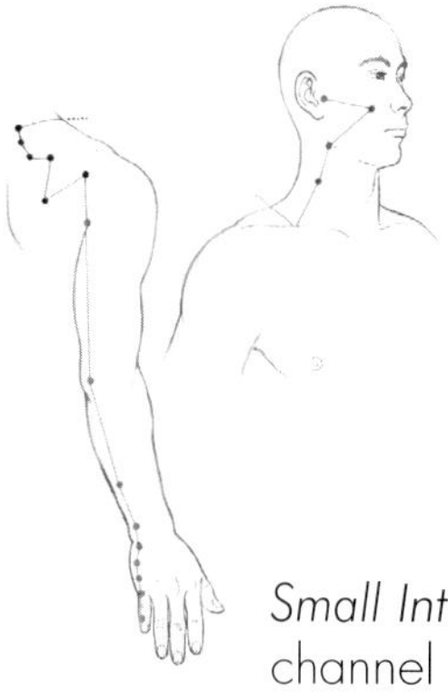

Small Intestine — Yang channel of Fire

The Fire element within our body, mind and emotions

Body

My Fire element shows itself in my face and on my tongue. The faculty of speech is a virtue of my Fire element, so I can become overtalkative, exuberant or even manic if my Fire imbalances. My fire can race out of control; if my spirit is agitated I can become hysterical. Slurring my words can indicate a displacement of my spirit.

Key tasks of my element involve the functions of my heart — the emperor. My Fire element moderates my internal organs through a special mechanism called *San Jiao*, meaning 'Three Burners'. This is a non-physical organ, which regulates my thorax, abdomen and urogenital system. It is like the office of the prime minister that oversees the carrying out of the will of the emperor. The prime minister is the pericardium which surrounds and protects the emperor. Just as a weak or isolated emperor can bring chaos to the land, the elements can become dysfunctional in the absence of sound leadership.

My Fire element is held in check by my Water element: this interaction influences the regularity of my heartbeat. Too much Fire will make my heart speed up and too little will slow it down. My heart circulates and governs my blood; it controls my blood vessels. Poor circulation, inflammations, swellings and bleeding all indicate a Fire imbalance. Vivid, panoramic dreams can also disclose an unsettled heart, especially when my dreams disturb my sleep.

Mind

In sharing my joyful spirit, all things around me are nourished. If I deny what my heart says I am fooled into thinking I am separate from the sea of consciousness that connects me with my surroundings. A poverty of spirit can turn my world into a lonely one. When I properly balance intuition with reason, my spirit will remain in connection with and support all the elements.

Emotions

My Fire element houses my spirit and resonates to the emotion of joy. I aspire to be trusting and empathetic; when I lovingly project these qualities, laughter fills the home.

Fear of betrayal can shroud my inner light and form a buttress against the outside world, affecting my ability to form deep relationships with those around me. When I feel safe and content, my bubbly nature is revealed and I will have a singsong lilt to my voice. This reflects also my relationship with *spleen* energy. (Earth element bestows the sound of song.)

Destiny of the Fire element

With reverence and love, I follow a path of authenticity and project a destiny of peace, joy and harmony. Through my supreme consciousness I master equanimity between the contracting nature of fear and the expansive qualities of joy and light.
I am in touch with my feelings. By extending love and gratitude, my gentle communion with the elements brings me joy.

In the pulse of our blood,
in the depths of our heart,
is our spirit to live and to love.

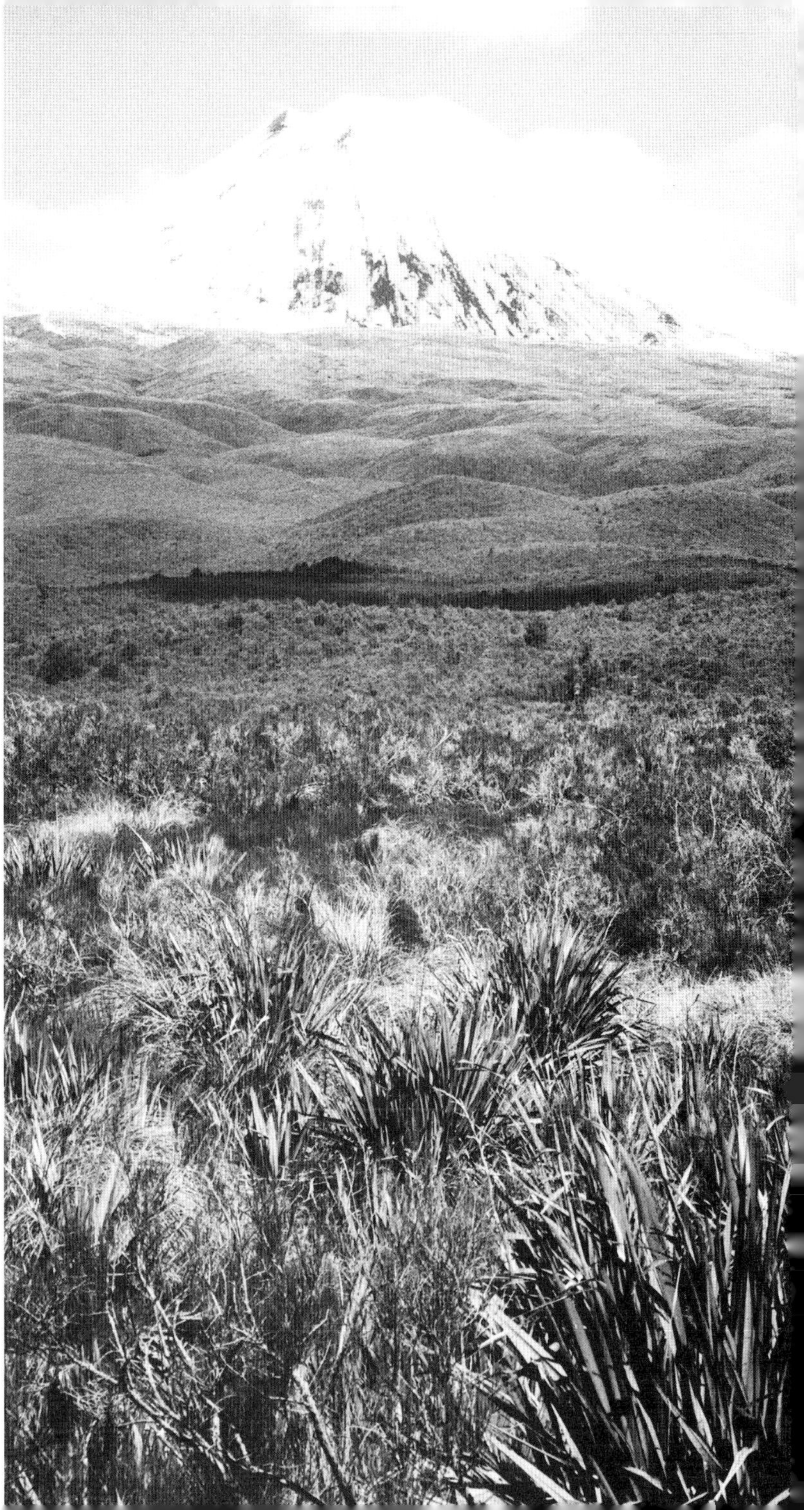

Harmony of the elements

Healing ourselves and each other

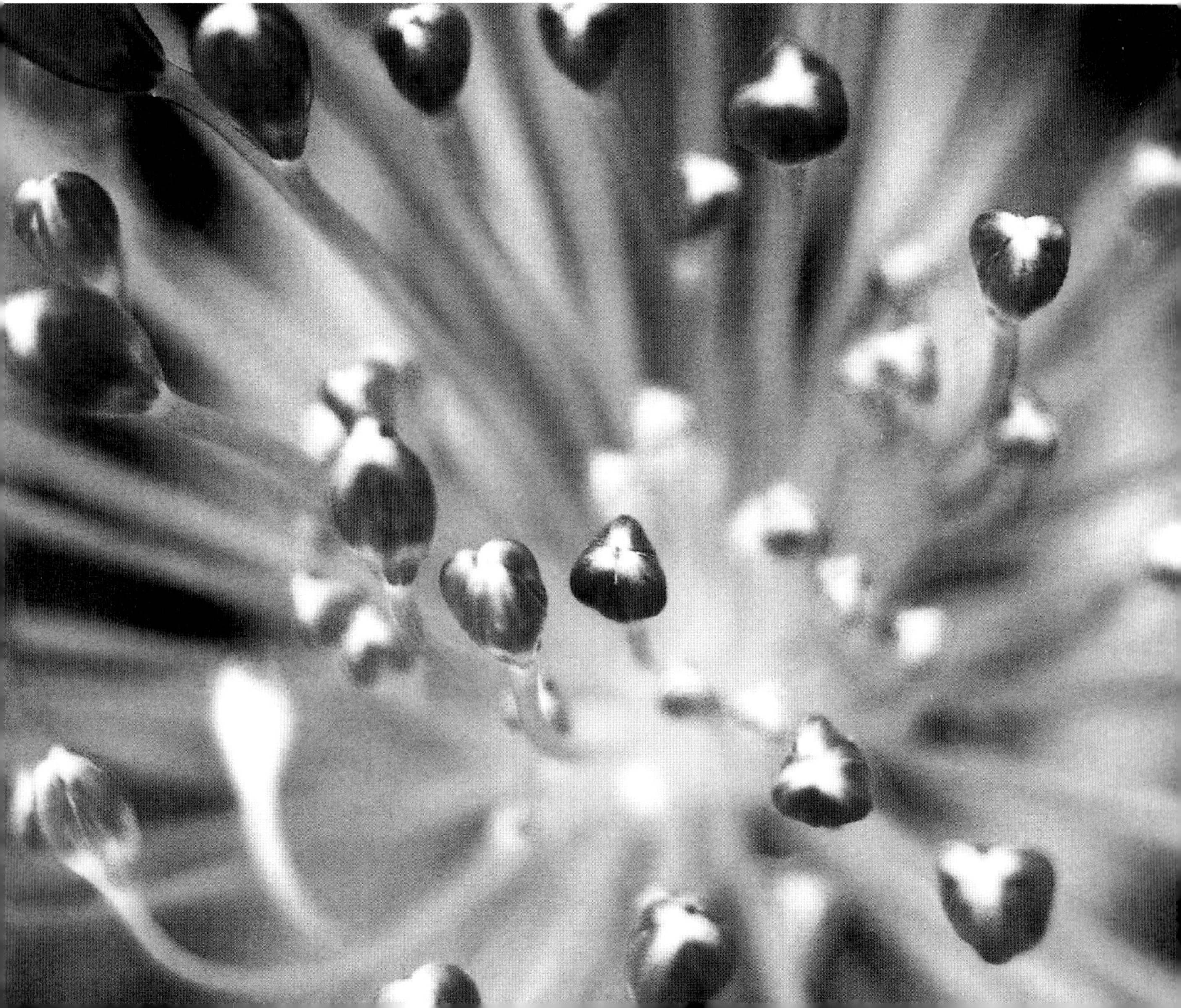

There is no matter independent of the smallest cell,
all matter is imbued with the presence of Qi.
Yin and Yang govern the moon and sun,
and exist within every aspect of creation.
The Five Elements are manifestations of nature;
a relationship between heaven and earth and all things between.

土 金 水 木 火

Moving together

We can marvel at the separate cells that make up the body of a bird, but only in their union do we see the beauty of a life.

Within every element are all of the Five Elements. Their separation is only an illusion we create so we can isolate each element for discussion. The elements swirl like coloured gases into each other, merging and moving like a great spinning nebula that constantly reveals new discoveries as we move through its form. There are no completely static reference points — the patterns change around us before our eyes. All of the elements are moving towards a certain state, but they never get 'there'. It is the movement of the elements that matters: the destiny, not the destination. In Five Element theory there is no completion to the creative journey and no separation of the journey's participants.

Every attribute of an element is also an attribute, in some way, of every other element. What is 'red' without any other colours or an object to carry the colour? What is a lung organ without a body that needs air? The Five Element theory perceives individuals within relationships, not individuals as lone entities, and these relationships have endless layers of interaction to explore.

We can look at our life — our body, emotions, spirit and 'soul-life' — and marvel at the interplay of the elements within us. What is 'true of us' is always less true in another light; what is 'fact' about our state of being is already shifting. Even our cells are being renewed every second.

Practitioners of many forms of healing use Five Element theory as a device for assessing the dispositions, tendencies, imbalances and characteristics of their clients. However, we humans are always more than the sum of our parts; each time we look at anyone or anything through the portal of the Five Element system, we must look afresh.

Destiny is the consciousness of motion;
emotion is that movement personified;
healing is love.

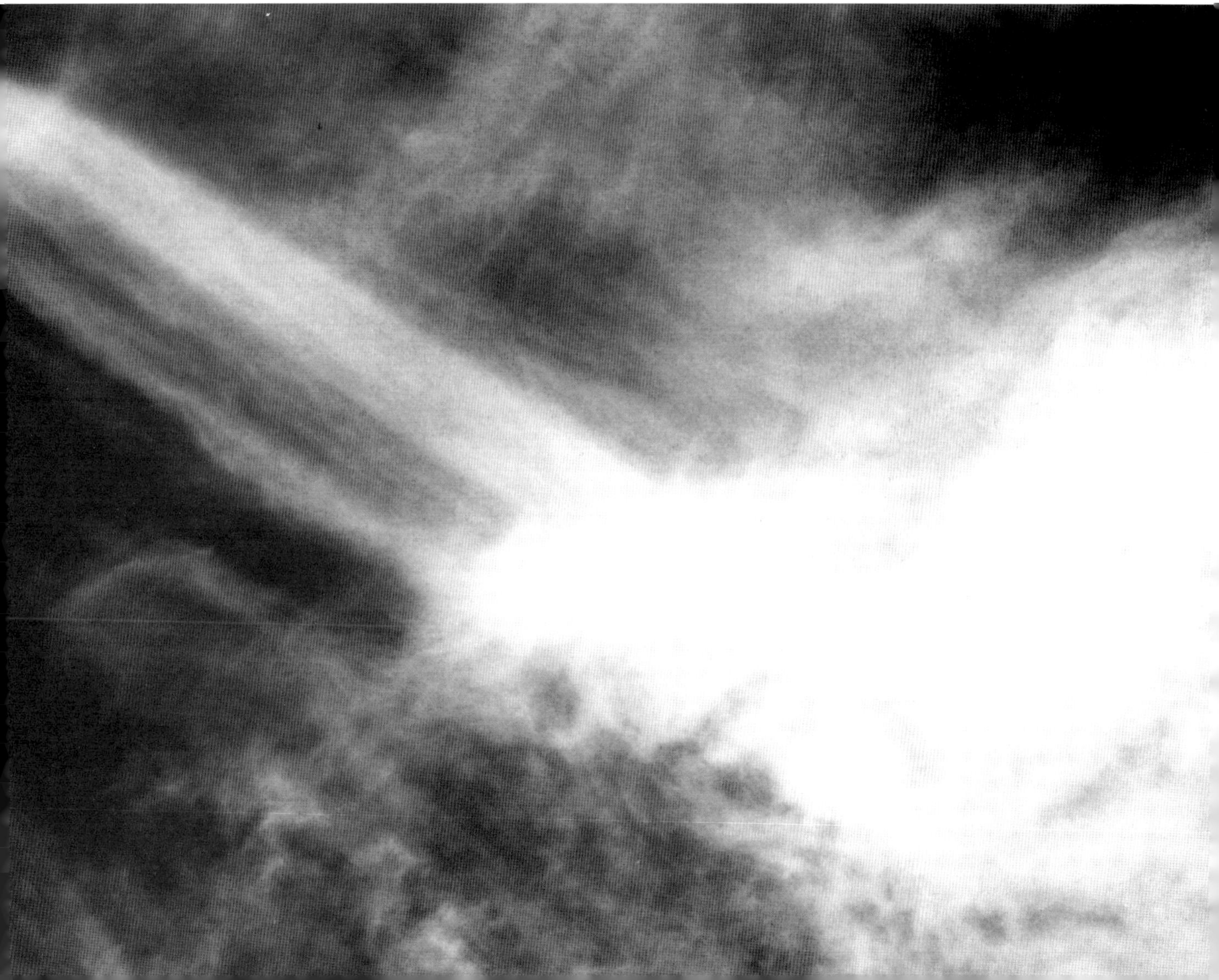

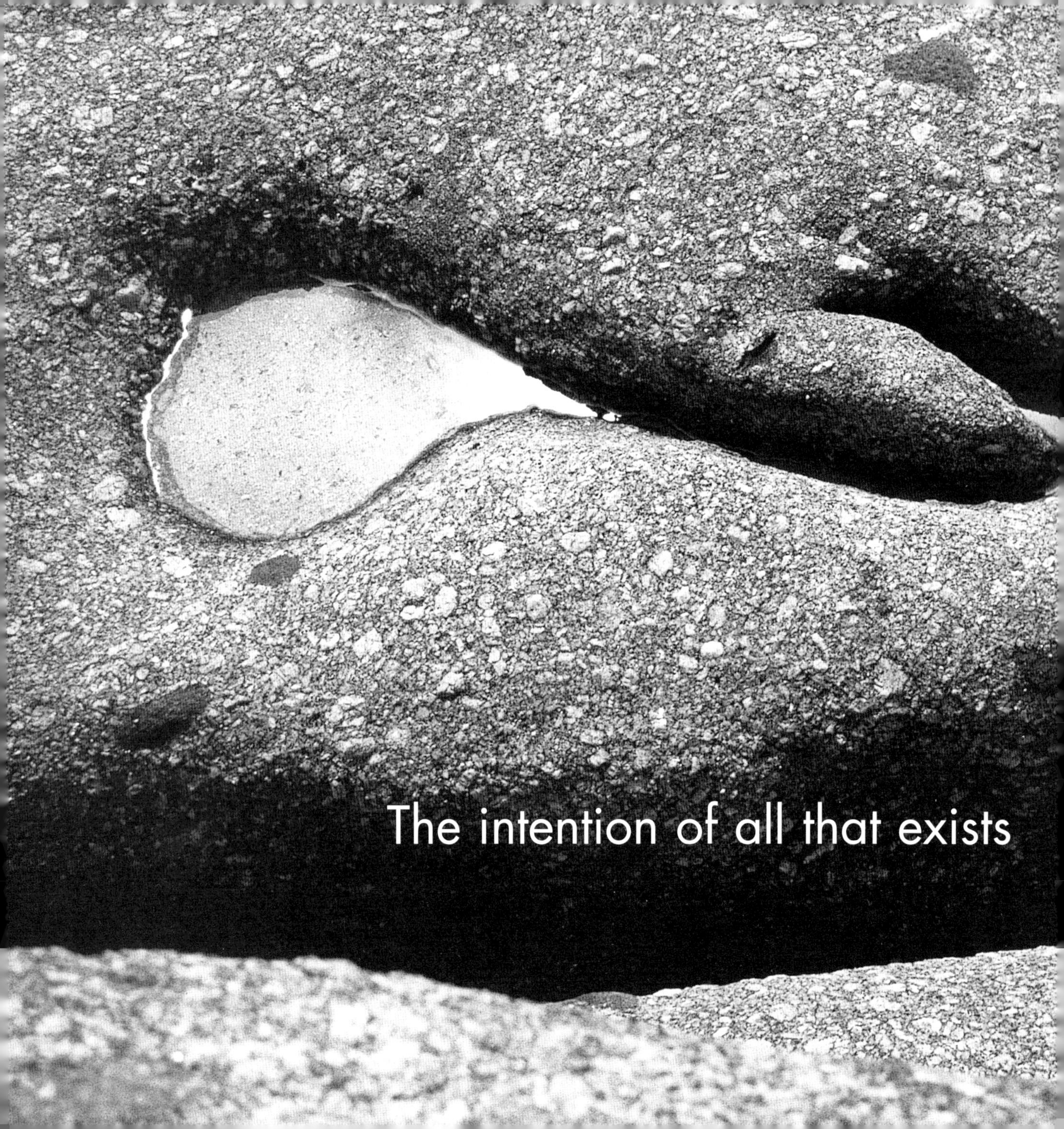
The intention of all that exists

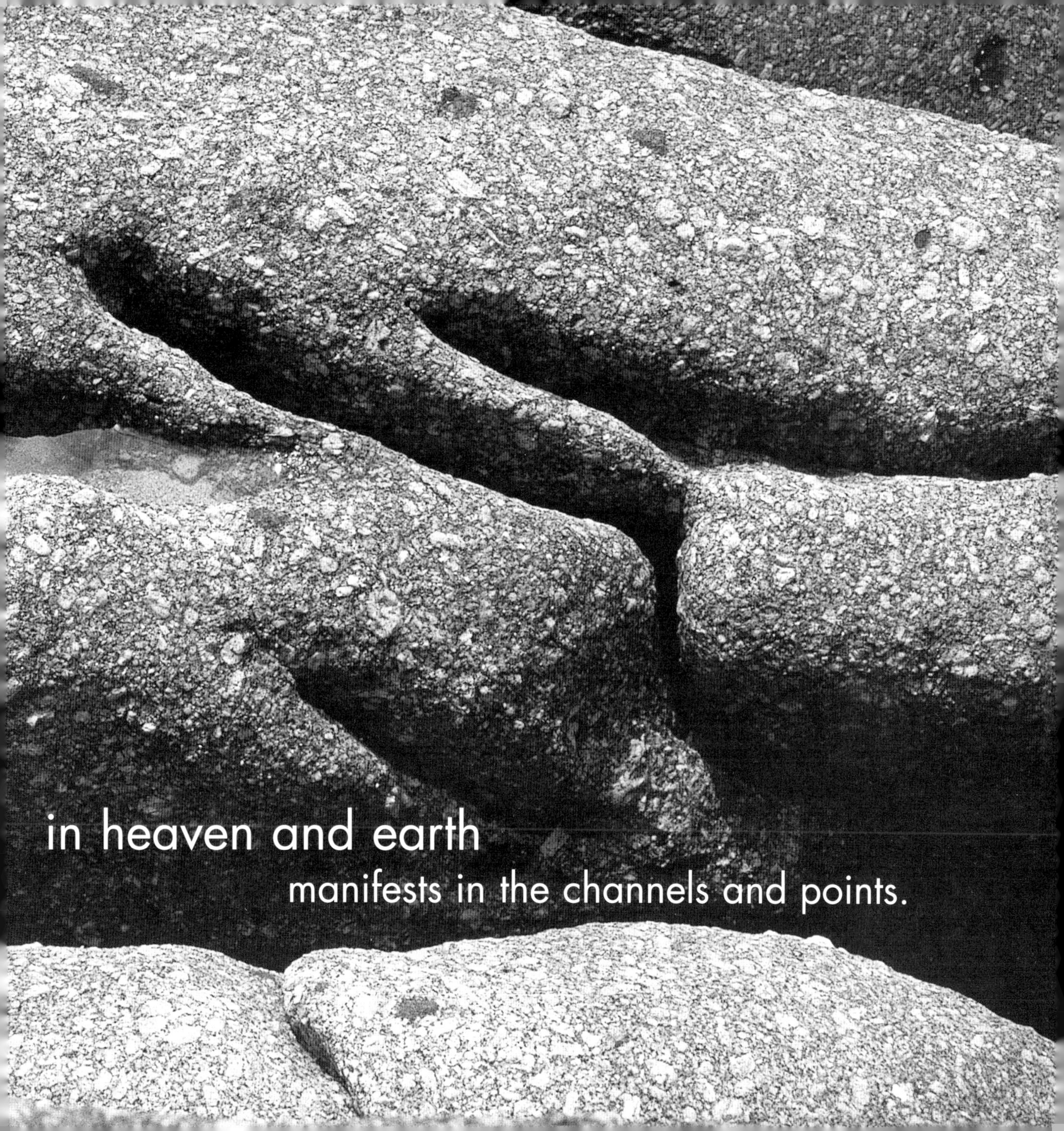

in heaven and earth
manifests in the channels and points.

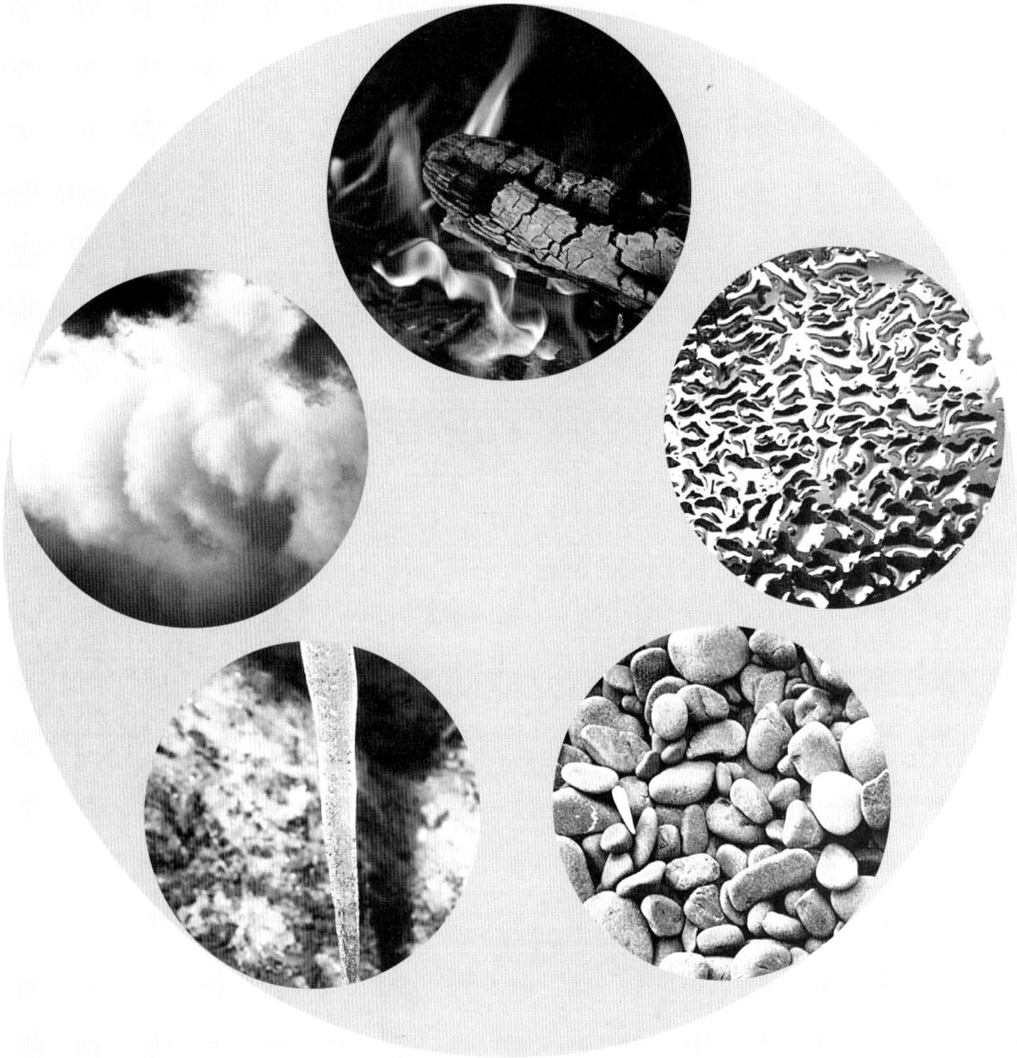

The climates and the organs

In Traditional Chinese Medicine particular interest is shown in conditions that are affected by the *climates*, or are the result of their influences. The names given to these climatic influences borrow their imagery from nature and can manifest from within, or have external origins. They are called *Wind, Damp, Cold, Dryness* and *Heat*.

These titles describe the energetic quality of each influence — the specific type of Qi — rather than just the literal phenomenon of each climatic occurrence in nature. However, the actual weather patterns can exasperate or relieve specific conditions, and sensitivity to weather changes can indicate what kind of influence is present in the body. As a reflection of the macrocosm, the body always strives to keep in balance with what is happening outside. A good example is a knee that always plays up before the rain, even when we are warm and dry. This will tell a practitioner of Traditional Chinese Medicine that there is dampness blocking the energy channels in the knee, and indicate which treatment is the most suitable to remove it.

Our bodies respond to the influences of the climates in notable patterns, and Traditional Chinese Medicine has correlated these tendencies to see which climatic influences affect which of the organs and channels. It is important to remember that the organs are not understood as separate mechanical features; they are identified by how they produce and distribute Qi and by what effect they have on the interactive functions that occur in our bodies. Each organ has its own particular manifestation of Qi — *spleen* Qi, *heart* Qi, *bladder* Qi and so on — and each climatic influence tends to be injurious to particular functions in our bodies:

Heat can be injurious to the *heart*,
Humidity and Damp to the *spleen*,
Cold to the *kidneys*,
Dryness to the *lungs*,
and Wind to the *liver*.

An understanding of these influences is not simple; an accurate diagnosis comes with many years of study of Traditional Chinese Medicine. While we needn't run inside to escape the sun for fear it will injure our heart, we must consider extreme conditions of any sort cautiously. Common sense can aid us in maintaining our health.

Traditionally, Wind is considered to be the harbinger of all disease from outside the body, and ridding the channels of this influence is a treatment principle for practitioners of Traditional Chinese Medicine. Wind can also be generated internally through damage to the cooling aspects of the body. A loss of cold leaves an excess of heat, as if we have turned down the cold water tap in the shower. This heat then causes the Qi to run rampant, like the wavy effect fire has on the air directly over it. This Wind generally moves upwards, causing such things as dizziness, headaches and ringing in the ears.

As with all systems in the Five Element theory, the climates are inseparably interactive. Together they complete the harmony of health.

Climates of the Five Elements

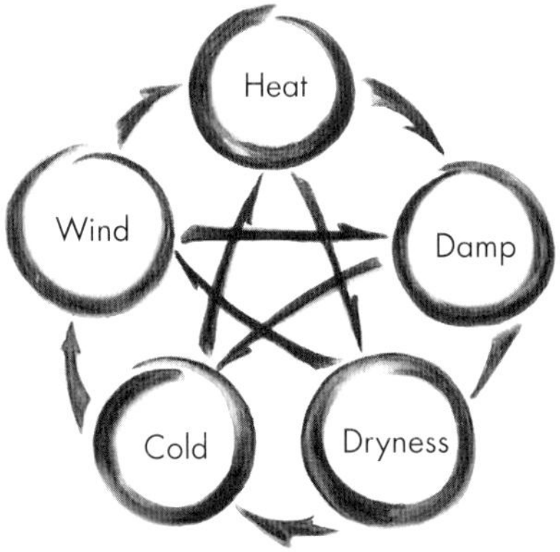

The body clock in Traditional Chinese Medicine

In Five Element theory the channels and organs associated with each element have predominant times of peak activity. Together, they complete a harmonious 24-hour cycle. People often prefer certain times of the day, or lack energy at other times. Patterns may point to imbalances due to either an elemental lack or an overabundance of a particular energy within our bodies. For example, people who wake up at 2.00 a.m. every morning might look to their Wood element as this is the time when Wood Qi is most active. These people may have excessive amounts of *liver* Qi. Similarly, people who fall asleep at around 6.00 p.m. every day may suspect they have low *kidney* Qi levels, as this is the time when *kidney* Qi is most active. Naturally, everyone's cycle is unique and the organ clock is only ever a guide that helps us add one piece to a much larger puzzle.

Time	Channel	Element
3.00 a.m. – 5.00 a.m.	*lung*	Metal
5.00 a.m. – 7.00 a.m.	*large intestine*	Metal
7.00 a.m. – 9.00 a.m.	*stomach*	Earth
9.00 a.m. – 11.00 a.m.	*spleen*	Earth
11.00 a.m. –1.00 p.m.	*heart*	Fire
1.00 p.m. – 3.00 p.m.	*small intestine*	Fire
3.00 p.m. – 5.00 p.m.	*bladder*	Water
5.00 p.m. – 7.00 p.m.	*kidney*	Water
7.00 p.m. – 9.00 p.m.	*pericardium*	Fire
9.00 p.m. – 11.00 p.m.	*three burners*	Fire
11.00 p.m. –1.00 a.m.	*gall bladder*	Wood
1.00 a.m. – 3.00 a.m.	*liver*	Wood

The five ages of our life

The philosophy of Five Element theory moves freely between things large and things small, and recognises repeating patterns between the macrocosm and the microcosm. A nautilus shell held in the palm of our hand may echo the forms we see in the body of an enormous nebula. When we look at an atomic particle through an electron microscope we may be reminded of the orbiting heavenly bodies as seen through an astronomical telescope. Time also reveals repeating patterns across different time frames. The 24-hour body clock illustrates the Five Element cycle we experience in the course of one day, but we also see a subtler long-term pattern reveal itself over a lifetime. By attributing loosely bracketed age groups to each of the elements we gain a non-traditional overview of energetic activity that echoes the flow of the Five Elements.

Water

Black — dawn, and the darkness whispers to the light

Preconception and birth

Primal forces stir in the depths of a pool as 'death' makes its transition into life in an embryonic world. The waters break and a human learns to use its body in a world of relative separation. This is an age when we are forming.

Wood

Green — early and mid morning; sharp light awakens change

Infancy to early teens

This is the coming of age — a time of promise and potential. The rebel flexes muscle, knows idealism, angers, exuberates. Life is rapid and raw. We are green and supple, and experience the power of growth.

Fire

Red — the heat of the day; the sun is in full expression

Early adult to mid life

The house is being built and the people gather together. This is a time of action, filled with the joy of living and the need to create and procreate. We enjoy the boldness of red and the heat of our blood.

Earth

Yellow — late afternoon and the light softens; shadows form

Mid to later life

The soft afternoon sun shines on our faces. We have knowledge of the world and will stow provisions to see us through the next age. Now is a time of mature fruition and the steadying of our life's focus. There are many things to be done, but still we have time to relax and enjoy good food and the comfort of home.

Metal

White — evening descends and the night brings quiet and peace

Older age to death

An objective awareness in our nature comes forward as the day starts to close. This is a time of quiet contentment and far-sighted thought processes; we attain the gift of 'overview'. Physical power diminishes and the spirit comes forward to welcome the coming of the night. We are retiring from worldly affairs; our bodies pale and harden. We are wizened, and know wisdom.

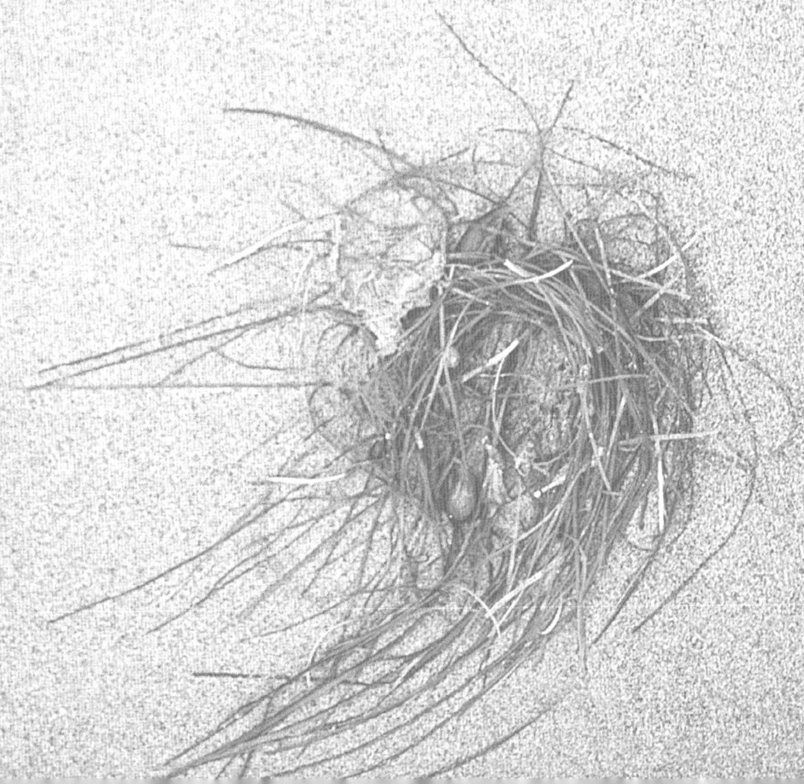

The five gestures of the elements

The Sheng construction cycle acknowledges five specific 'gestures' or 'intentions', each belonging to one of the elements, that are aspects of creation and expressions of the movement of life. These gestures are the energetic directions — the destiny — in which each element aspires to move. Together these directions help us to visualise the Five Elements in motion and demonstrate the dynamics of elemental interaction.

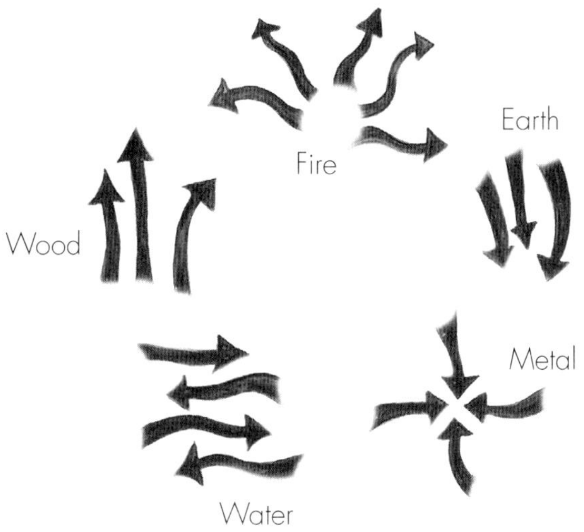

Fire travels outwards;
Earth centralises;
Metal condenses;
Water flows;
Wood aspires upwards.

Food and the Five Elements

In Traditional Chinese Medicine, food is grouped into Yin or Yang and five distinct flavours: sour, bitter, sweet, pungent and salty. Each of these has a distinct healing effect. Each of these food groups breaks down into five types of grain, domestic animal, vegetable and fruit. All of these have relative qualities of Yin and Yang, and all of them relate to particular elements and their associated organs.

Wood has the **sour** taste, which affects the liver.
Fire has the **bitter** taste, which affects the heart.
Earth has the **sweet** taste, which affects the spleen.
Metal has the **pungent** taste, which affects the lung.
Water has the **salty** taste, which affects the kidneys.

The individual organs benefit from small quantities of these specific flavours and are harmed by excess quantities. The way a food is prepared also changes the way it affects our bodies. Frying, boiling and roasting, for instance, all have different effects on the healing powers of food.

In Five Element theory foods are grouped by their energetic properties and their proven ability to restore internal balance. The Five Element categories recognise the need for variety and biodiversity and ensure that every element is represented in a healthy diet.

Food is also categorised by colour, texture, growing method, direction of growth, season of growth, density of matter and environment of occurrence. Some foods, like some other element associations, seem logical in their categorisation: a bright red pepper grown in the heat of summer is a Fire food, while sweet yellow honey collected in the lazy days of late summer is a strong Earth food. If a natural food menu includes plenty of colour, a variety of cooking methods, tastes and textures, it is likely to be balanced with the energetic qualities of the Five Elements.

In Traditional Chinese Medicine food is considered to be a primary medicine. It is approached with both a metaphysical and physical logic — a blend of observation, intuition and proven experience. Food feeds our body, mind, emotions and spirit by balancing Yin and Yang and the Five Elements.

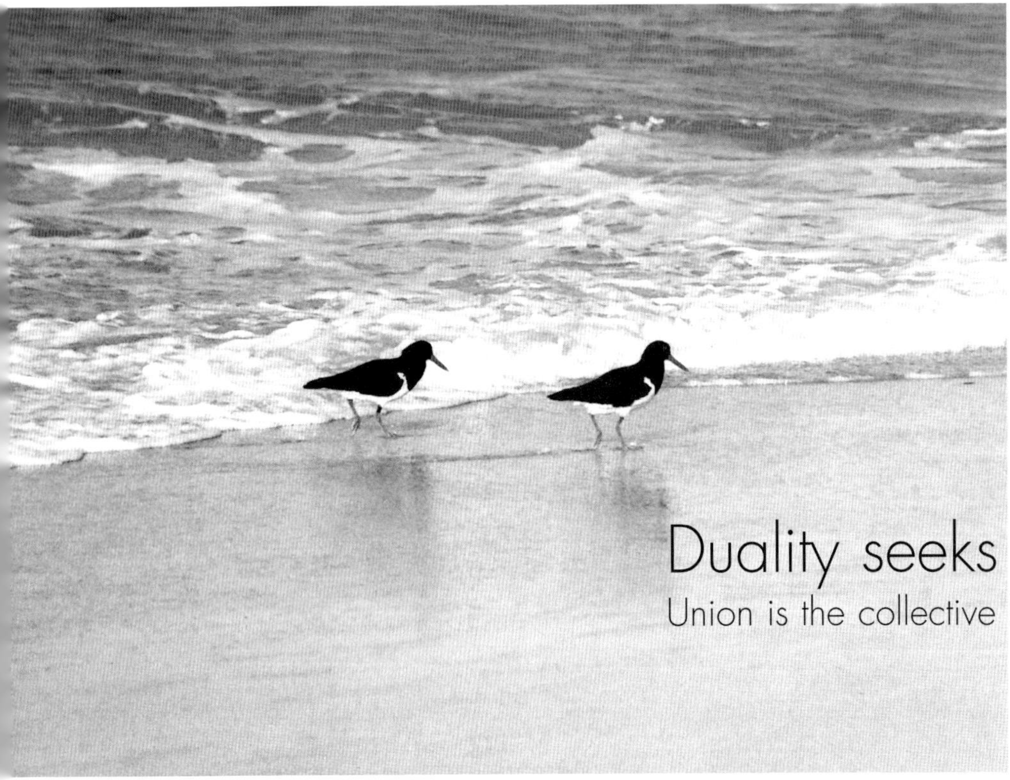

Duality seeks union.

Union is the collective harmony of duality.

Duality and union: the forces of creation

Humans are not separate from this planet.
The elements are not unto themselves;
each relies, accommodates and becomes the other —
woman and man are one.

Duality and union are the qualities that give life to the Five Elements and to all worldly phenomena. In birth we begin our discovery of duality and physical separation. We move from a world of darkness into a world of light, from the encompassing embryonic fluid into the relatively dry atmosphere of our planet. In time we learn of the duality of heaven and earth, of hot and cold, day and night, hard and soft, and even of death and life. We discover that Yin and Yang are not one, but neither are they two. Harmony exists only because of the interaction of differing phenomena.

In human sexual reproduction we connect with the primary oneness of union from which all life stems. Although physical life cannot exist without the union of complementary forces, no life exists as a complete or unchanging union of these opposites. Duality constantly seeks union, and harmony is the result of dualism achieving equilibrium — albeit ever-changing equilibrium. At the moment sperm and egg merge in perfect union they are already causing cells to divide in order to build a body of flesh. This body becomes identifiable as 'separate' from the world around it and we are able to name a new being.

Traditional Chinese Medicine works closely with the concept of Yin and Yang. To imagine the end of complementary and antagonistic forces is to imagine a lifeless world and a human body with no Qi and no pulse. The practitioner who understands Yin and Yang will strive to create healthy balances of Qi, where no one force exerts dominance over another; but they will also understand that life exists as a creative dance that is in constant motion. Healing, like the Five Elements, is always a flowing process of change.

The central element

The Five Element theory is sometimes illustrated in a schematic that shows four elements around the fifth element, the Earth — Mother Earth. In this schematic, Earth acts as a reference point or hub for the other elements and is a place where all the other elements can be balanced by using the qualities of contemplation, mindfulness and compassion.

Earth stands at the centre of our emotional being. When we are angry (Wood), depressed (Metal), joyous (Fire), or frightened (Water), we can come back to our centre and acknowledge the emotion from a stable viewpoint. This is like standing in the eye of a storm; everything is observed and is 'played out', but the ground where we stand remains calm and the 'home' remains intact.

The Central Earth system

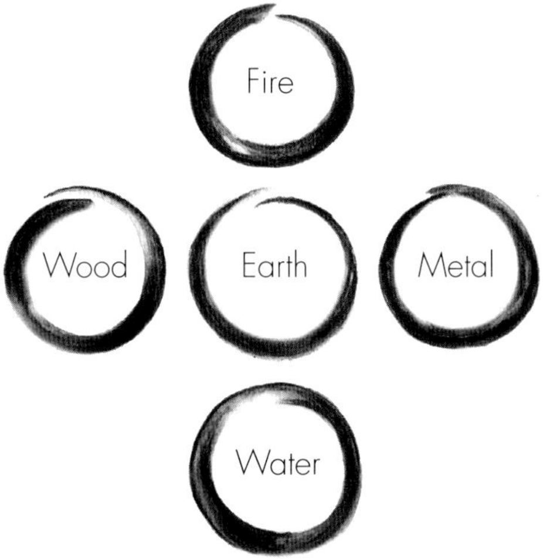

Zen Shiatsu is a meditative form of body work from Japan. It teaches that the primary diagnostic and treatment area for the Earth element is at the centre of the abdomen, around the navel. Zen Shiatsu practitioners begin a session by placing their hands on the *Hara* of their client. A hand resting on a belly is incredibly comforting and nurturing, as a mother calming a baby knows. To touch a person's *Hara* requires respect (mindfulness) from the giver and trust (permission) from the receiver. Zen Shiatsu recognises that this is a sacred place where healing can occur.

The sage sits in the
eye of the storm.
The mind does not
follow the wind.

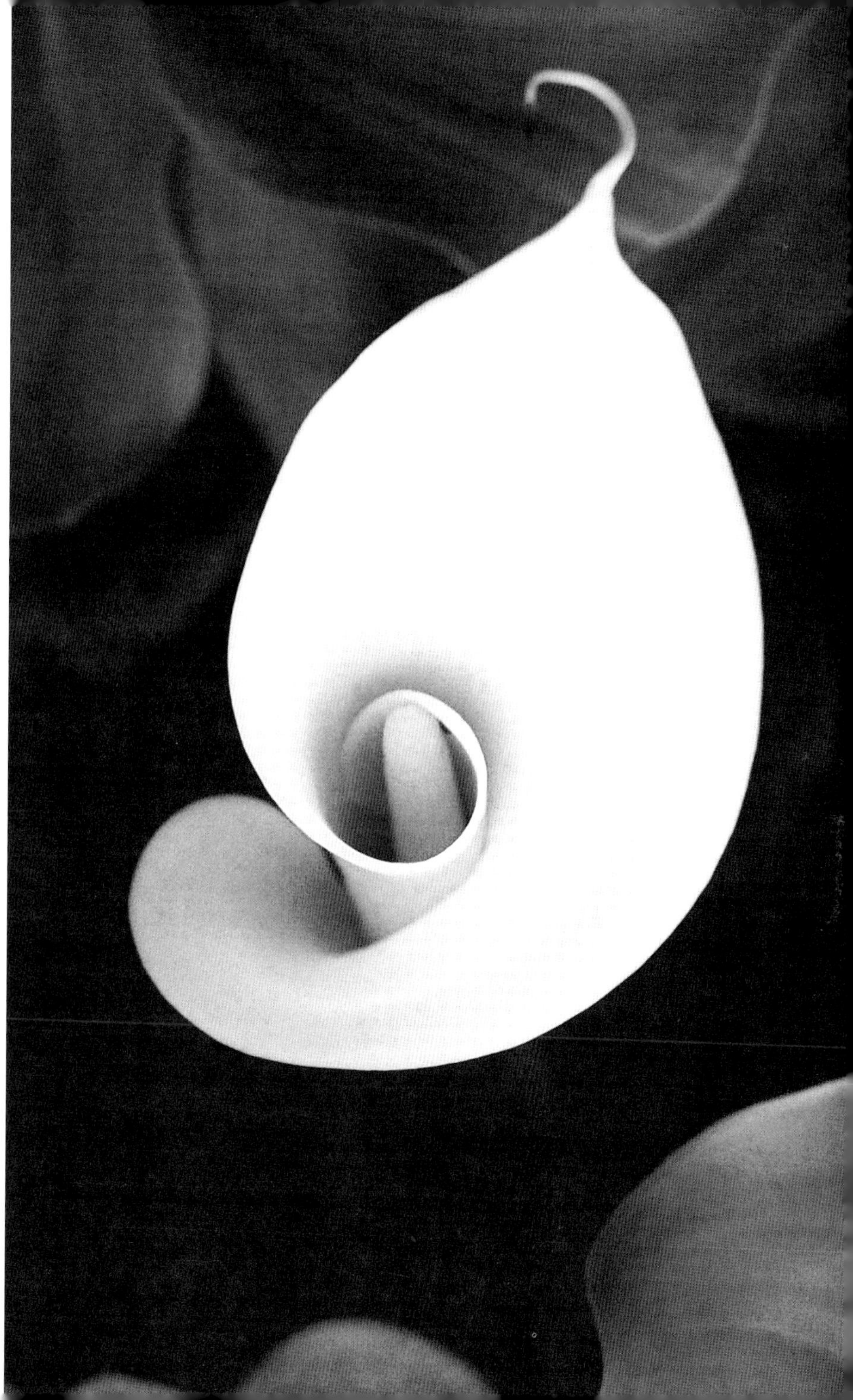

The healer is a mirror,
causing reflections on our true nature.

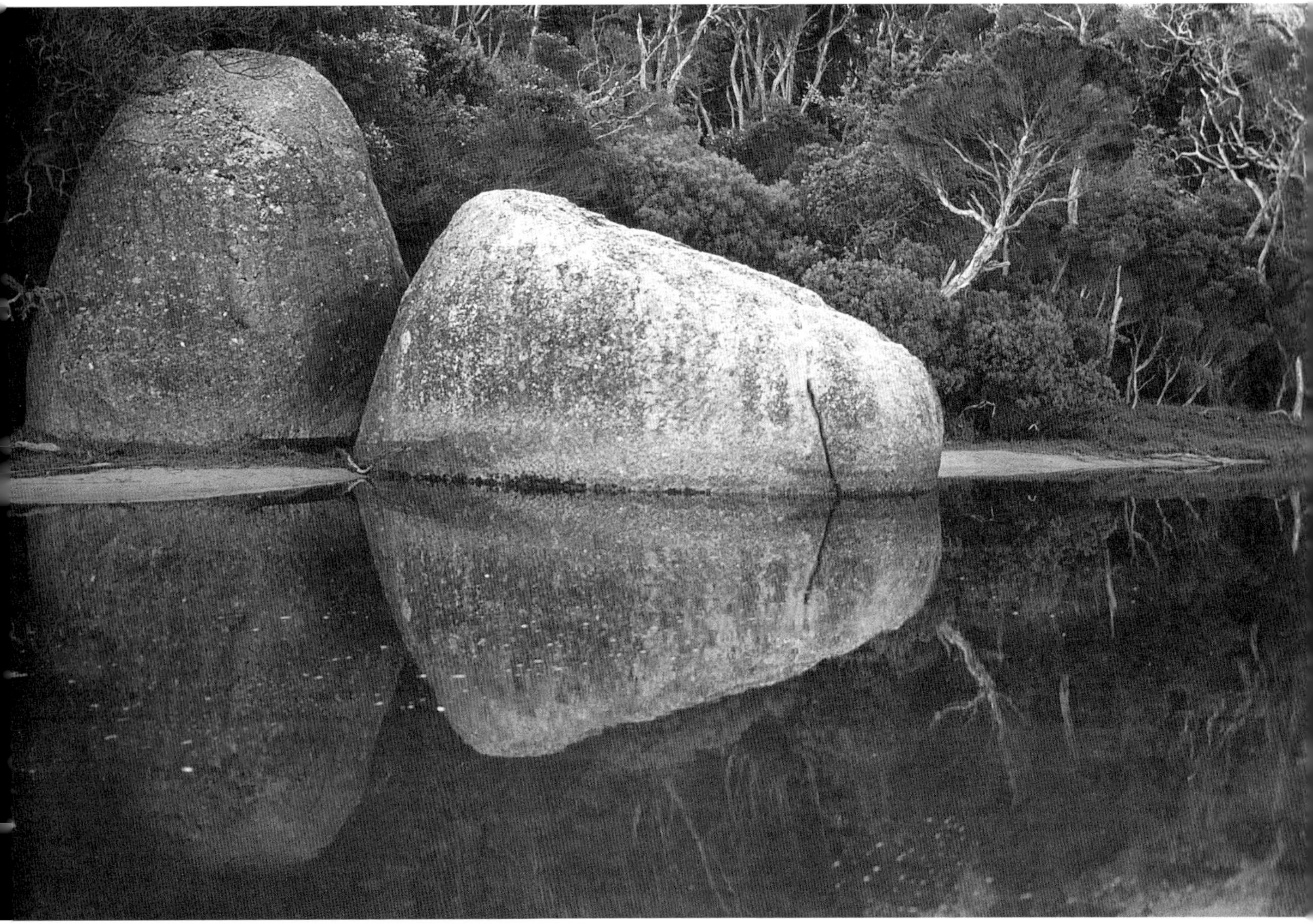

Dan Tien: the centre of our being

Martial arts such as Aikido and Tai Chi and healing arts such as Reiki and Qi Gong teach that there is a gathering place for Qi located below our navel, centred in our *Hara*. In Traditional Chinese Medicine this is called *Dan Tien* (*Tanden* in Japanese, *Dan Jeon* in Korean). There are actually two more of these Qi generation and storage areas in our bodies; one between the eyebrows and one in the solar plexus, but the term is usually used to refer to *Dan Tien* in the lower *Hara* — the centre of our being. *Dan Tien* is the focus of attention in many Asian practices, of which Qi Gong and Aikido are good examples.

Qi Gong

Qi Gong (also Chi Kung) is a practice that uses postures, meditation and breath exercises to enhance Qi flow and well-being. Most Qi Gong styles encourage awareness of *Dan Tien* and use visualisations that focus our attention on this Qi centre. This allows us to feel 'grounded' and balanced, and to move with economy and ease. Qi Gong exercises are aimed to enhance specific aspects of our body, mind and spirit by increasing the flow of Qi in the channels; a posture might be especially good for raising *lung* Qi or for stimulating *liver* Qi. Energising *Dan Tien* is beneficial to our whole system and can have a particularly strong effect on our *kidney* Qi.

Aikido

While acknowledging a four element system based on Shinto beliefs, Japanese Aikido shares the same understanding of Qi (Ki) and *Dan Tien* as Traditional Chinese Medicine. Sensei Tohei, the founder of 'Ki Society Aikido', taught that 'keeping *one-point*' was the first of four principles used in Aikido to unify body and mind. *One-point* is another name for lower *Dan Tien*. Keeping an awareness of *Dan Tien* allows Aikido masters to remain immensely stable, physically, mentally and spiritually, even in a chaotic environment. It is very difficult to unbalance someone who has a strong *one-point* and a good understanding of Ki (Qi) flow. At the age of eighty the founder of Aikido, Morihei Ueshiba (O' Sensei) could not be caught off-balance and could repel a group of 'attackers', sending them to the dojo floor, with little apparent effort.

In meditation, whether sitting or moving, we can use our breath to enliven *Dan Tien* and to still the chatter of our mind, becoming mindful of the present. Our thoughts are clarified and we experience the dynamic calm of being centred.

Dan Tien meditation

(Allow yourself 20 minutes for this meditation.)

Sit comfortably in your meditation posture. Let your mind follow the movements of your breath as it enters and exits gently through the nose. Your mouth is relaxed, lips closed, with your tongue resting on your upper palate. Your eyes are open and maintain a soft focus on the ground about three feet from where you sit. Your spine is upright but not rigid and your shoulders are relaxed.

Bring your hands together just below the navel. Cup the right hand with the left, palms upward, and have an awareness of a point about a few centimetres below the navel, within the belly. This is your *Dan Tien*, the centre of your body. Allow your breath to fill your belly and circulate within and around *Dan Tien*.

Enjoy the space between the in-breath and the out-breath, and rest in the stillness of the one-point. Stay in your belly. If your thoughts wander, gently come back to following your breath. Don't judge your thoughts or fight against them — allow them to come as they will and leave again without being followed.

Stay in the belly. Feel the in-breath expand in *Dan Tien* and the out-breath flood your body with Qi. Feel the relaxation in your body while maintaining the awareness of being only here and 'now'.

Feel the stillness and completeness of this moment; be only here. Only now. This moment is imbued with dynamic ease. You are awake. This moment is you. You are not your thoughts.

Allow *Dan Tien* to be the centre of your Universe, a place of great peace that extends out to all beings. Stay with your meditation, stay with *Dan Tien*.

At the end of your meditation slowly begin to move first your fingers and toes. Look around at the world. In time, gently stand, moving from the one-point in your belly. Where first *Dan Tien* moves, the body follows.

During the day contemplate the word 'peace'.

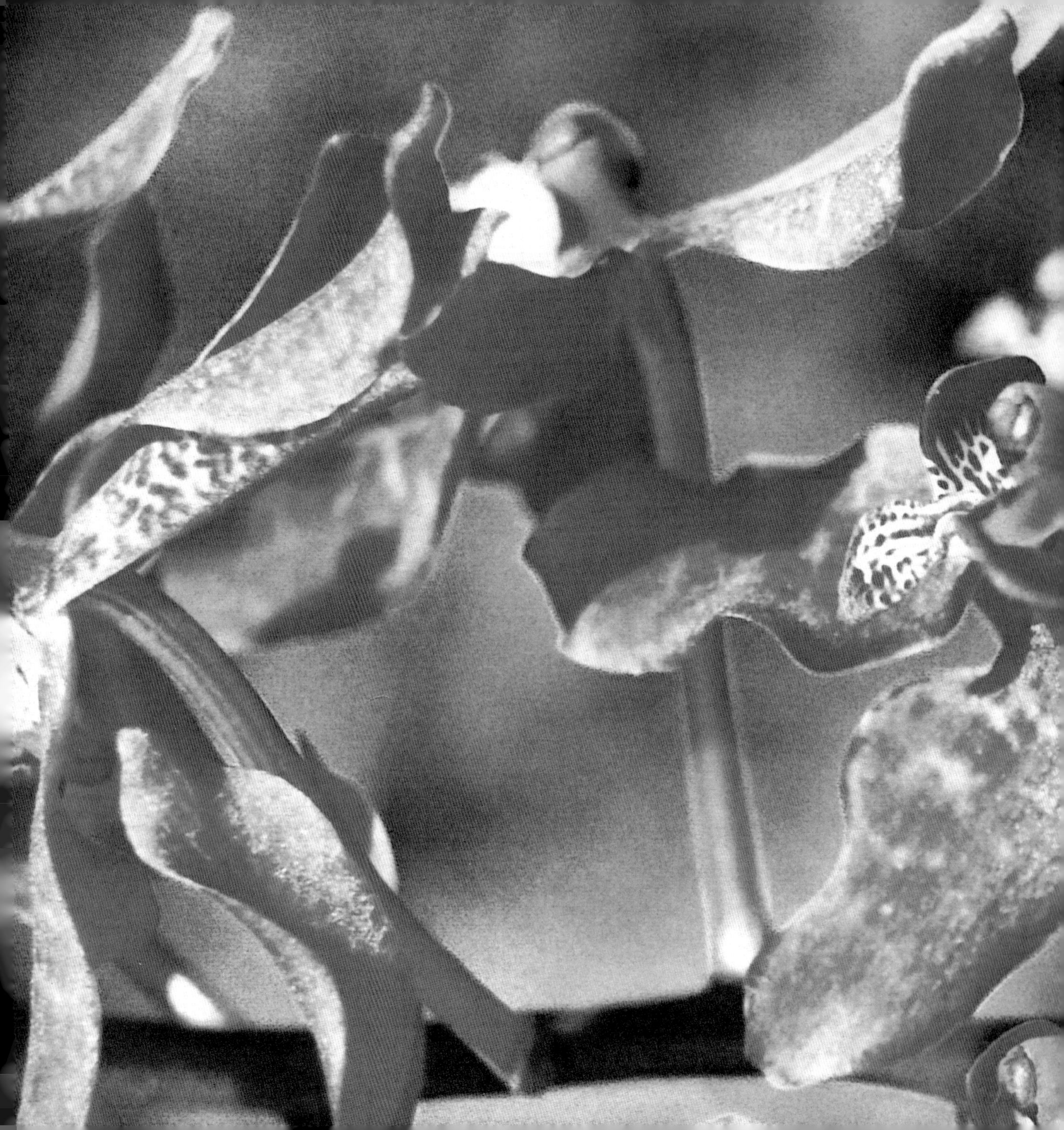

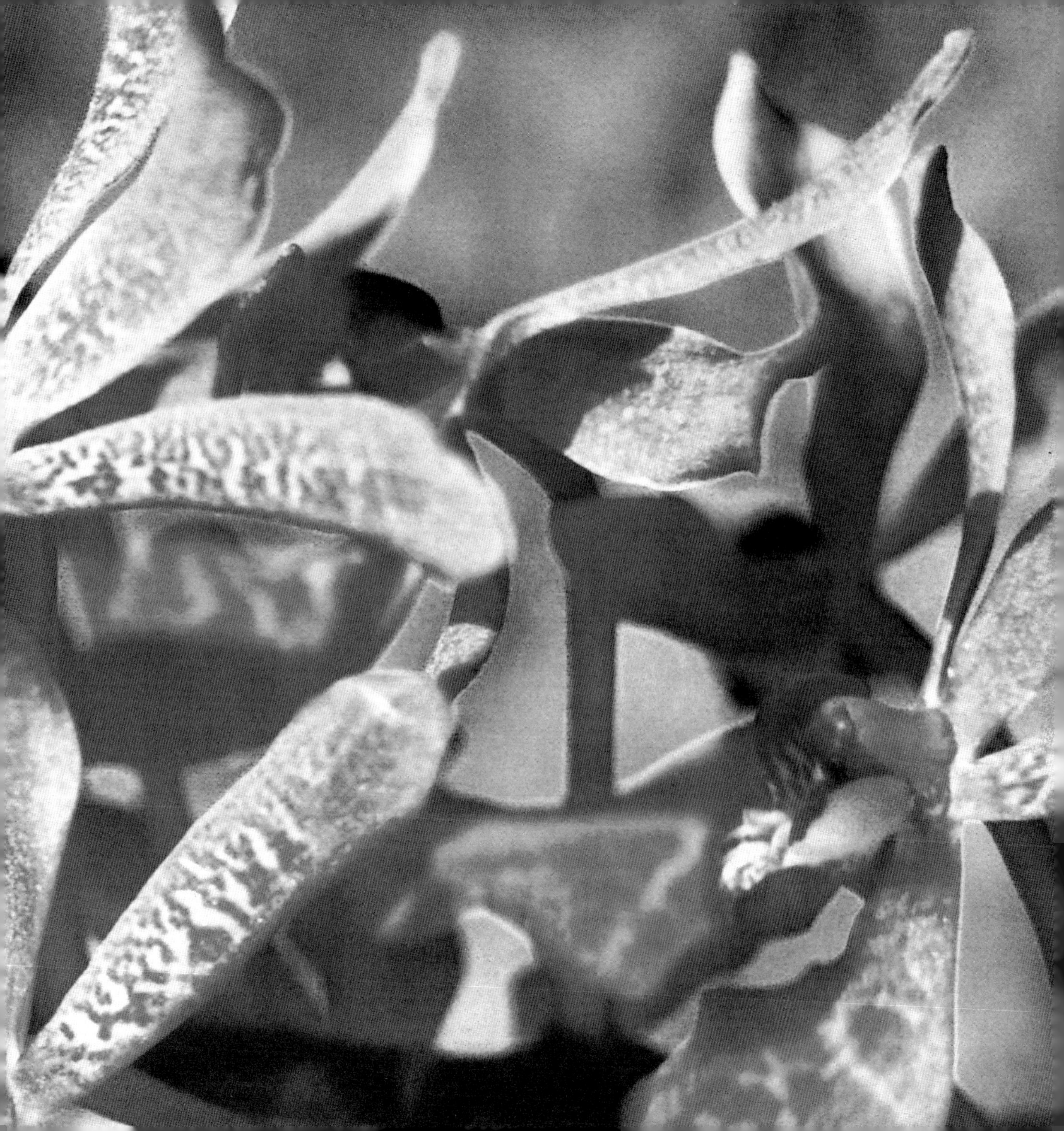

The spirit of our nature

We are the healers, and compassion is the fundamental principle in all healing. Compassion allows us to nurture ourselves as a natural act of living and to heal others as a natural act of love.

Preventative medicine is a major focus in Oriental philosophy. Traditional Chinese Medicine uses the Five Element theory as a tool for highlighting the signs that predispose a person to disease. We know that an imbalance in the flow of the elements has associated 'telltale' attributes and that by recognising these signs we can ward away illness both within our own lives and within our world.

The ancient Five Element theory derives from studying and understanding patterns developed over millennia in the natural world. By respecting these patterns we are able to heal states of imbalance and find harmony in our lives.

We are an extraordinary part of the Spirit of Nature.

土 金 水 木 火

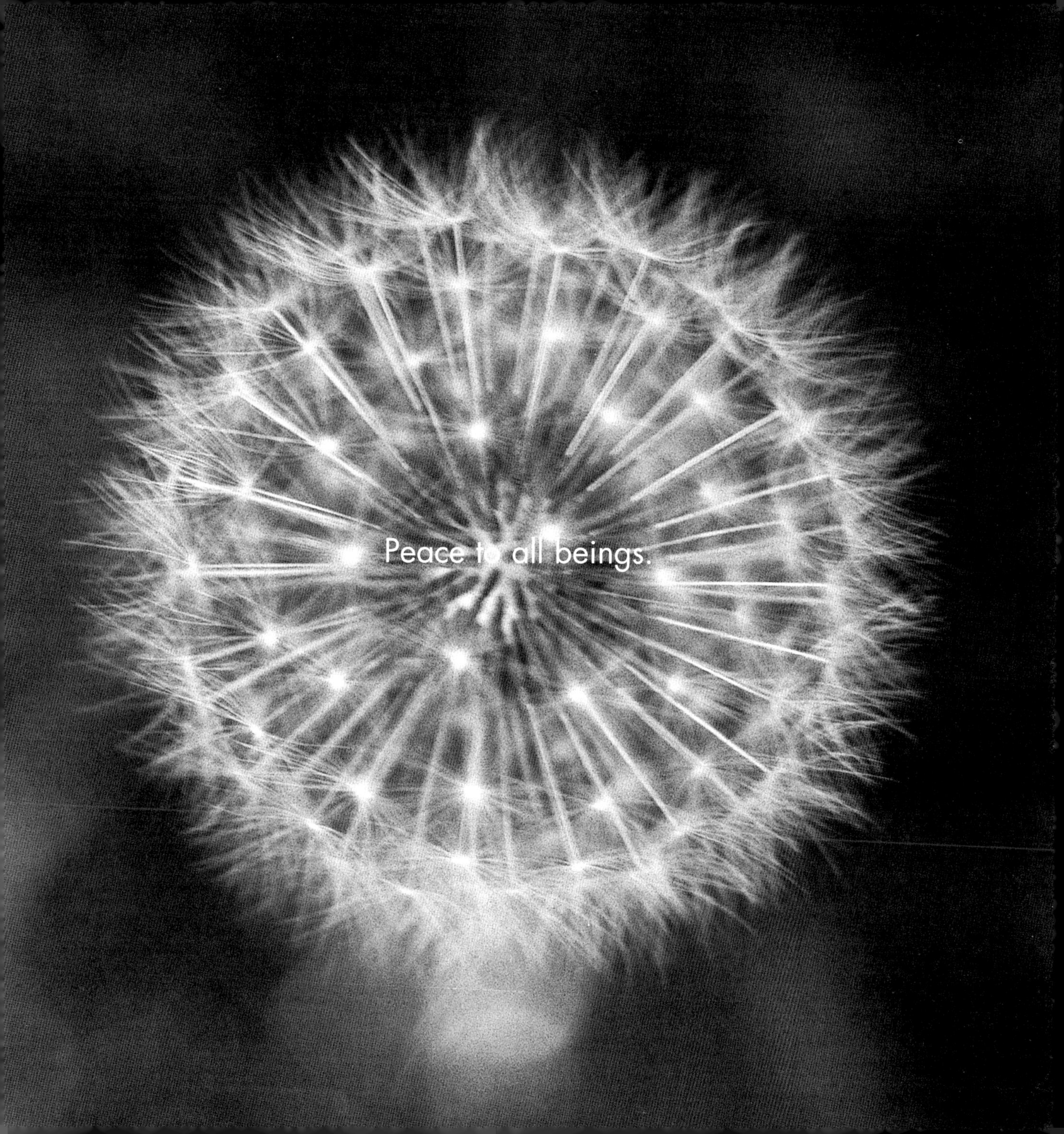
Peace to all beings.

Glossary

Acupressure Healing using points, as in acupuncture, but not needles. Pressure is applied to the points, often with the thumbs, fingers or other implements, to promote healthy Qi flow.

Aikido Japanese martial art developed by Morihei Ueshiba that promotes harmonising of Ki. Aikido is a discipline concerned with peaceful resolution of conflict.

Ampuku Diagnosis and treatment of the *Hara*, and consequently of the whole person. In Zen Shiatsu the Hara is schematically divided into areas that each relate to specific channels, which can be balanced with palpation and massage.

Ayurvedic Traditional Hindu medical system that includes breathing exercises, diet and herbs, and philosophies designed to restore and maintain the natural balances in our body systems.

Baihui A special point (Du 20) located on the top of the head, in Traditional Chinese Medicine.

Channels Refers to the flow of Qi as mapped by practitioners of Traditional Chinese Medicine. Sometimes called meridians, these are the networks by which Qi moves throughout the body.

Chi Alternative (older) spelling of Qi.

Chi Kung Alternative spelling of Qi Gong.

Ch'an (Chuan) The Chinese word for Zen.

Confucianism The study and practice of the teachings of Confucius (551–479 BCE), a famous Chinese philosopher who emphasised cultural order and etiquette.

Dadun A *liver* (Wood) channel point (Lv.1) in Traditional Chinese Medicine.

Dao Meaning the 'Way', the Chinese philosophy of 'oneness', or universalism. Sometimes spelt Tao.

Dao Te Ching A Chinese book dating to around 409 BCE that speaks poetically of the Dao. Written by a legendary figure named Lao Tzu.

Daoism The study of the Dao.

Dan Tien Point about 3cm below the navel and within the abdomen. *Dan Tien* is referred to in many practices as the physical centre of our being.

Do-in The stimulation of Qi in the channels and points through exercises and self-massage.

Dojo The practice room for Japanese martial arts.

Dualism The theory that there are always two great forces or principles at work. In relation to Yin and Yang, dualism describes the healthy interaction of opposites that together create harmony.

Feng Shui Meaning 'water, wind', the ancient Eastern art and science of creating balanced energy in an environment through acknowledgement of Five Element theory. True Feng Shui is a type of geomancy that acknowledges our need to live harmoniously in the natural world.

Gaohuangshu A *urinary bladder* (Water) point (U.B.43) in Traditional Chinese Medicine.

Hara Japanese word meaning 'belly', which is considered to be a sacred area of the body.

Hegu A *large intestine* (Metal) point (L.I.4) in Traditional Chinese Medicine.

Hun The Chinese word for soul, an active and integral part of our being.

In–Yo The Japanese words for Yin and Yang.

Ki The Japanese word for Qi.

Ko The control cycle of the Wu Xing, or Five Element interaction.

Lao Tzu Meaning 'Great Master', this title is attributed to the author of the *Dao Te Ching*.

Lieque A *lung* channel (Metal) point (Lu.7) in Traditional Chinese Medicine.

Makaho Exercises or 'meridian stretches' that are used and taught by Zen Shiatsu practitioners to promote good Ki flow.

Mahayana A tradition of Buddhism. From the Sanskrit words meaning 'great' (*maha*) and 'vehicle' (*yana*).

Meridians See channels.

Mindfulness The state of being completely present in this moment and attuned to the contemporary nature of life.

Moxibustion Traditional Chinese Medicine practice of applying heat, often created by burning mugwort. It is used either as a healing technique in itself or in combination with needles. The mugwort is usually dried and pressed into a stick that can be lit like a giant incense stick and held near a point that requires this type of treatment.

Neiguan A *pericardium* (Fire) channel point (Pc.6) in Traditional Chinese Medicine.

No mind A term sometimes used in Zen practice that describes life as it exists in the absence of excessive thought. It refers to the pure nature of immediacy and the simplicity of our being in the absence of affectation.

One-point A term used to describe *Dan Tien*.

Qi A Chinese word to describe 'life force'.

Qi Gong (Qigong) Health-giving Chinese exercises designed to stimulate specific channels and enhance the natural balances in our bodies of Yin and Yang, and Qi.

Qimen A *liver* (Wood) channel point (Lv.14) in Traditional Chinese Medicine.

Reiki A natural therapy from Japan, Reiki literally means 'universal' (*rei*), 'life force' (*ki*). Reiki practitioners may direct universal Ki to their subject rather than stimulate the Ki already present in their subject.

Ruah The Hebrew word for both 'wind' and 'spirit'.

Sanjiao Also called 'Three Burners' or 'Triple Heater'. This is a Fire element channel that does not have a physical organ associated with it.

Sanyinjiao A major *spleen* (Earth) channel point (Sp.6) in Traditional Chinese Medicine. It is also the meeting point for *spleen*, *kidney* and *liver* the three Yin channels found in the legs.

Sensei The Japanese term for teacher, used as a mark of respect in martial art Dojos.

Shaochong A *heart* (Fire) channel point (H.9) in Traditional Chinese Medicine.

Shaohai A *heart* (Fire) channel point (H.3) in Traditional Chinese Medicine.

Shen Shen is the Chinese term for 'the spirit'.

Shenmen A *heart* (Fire) channel point (H.7) in Traditional Chinese Medicine.

Shenshu A *urinary bladder* (Water) channel point (U.B.23) in Traditional Chinese Medicine.

Sheng The construction cycle of the Wu Xing, or Five Element schematic.

Shiatsu Literally meaning 'finger pressure', Shiatsu is a Japanese body therapy deriving from traditional Anma massage, Do-in, and Traditional Chinese Medicine. It involves acupressure, stretches, exercises and philosophies designed to balance Yin and Yang and harmonise Ki in the body. Among the many styles are two main schools: 'Zen' or 'Iokai' style, as taught by Shizuto Masunaga, and 'Namikoshi' style, as taught by Tokujiro Namikoshi. Also popular is 'Ohashiatsu' as taught by Wataru Ohashi and 'Healing Shiatsu' as taught by Sonia Moriceau.

Shinto The indigenous religion of Japan, pre-dating Buddhism.

Sumi-e A Japanese painting technique that is as much a meditation as an art form. The student typically paints with carefully prepared black ink onto rice paper using a soft, pointed brush. There are no second attempts, and each stroke becomes an act of mindfulness.

T'so Ch'an The Chinese term for *zazen*, a Zen practice involving sitting meditation.

Tai Chi A health-giving Chinese martial art that promotes and draws upon Qi flow in the body.

Taichong A *liver* (Wood) channel point (Lv. 3) in Traditional Chinese Medicine.

Taixi A *kidney* (Water) channel point (K.3) in Traditional Chinese Medicine.

Taiyuan A *lung* channel (Metal) point (Lu.9) in Traditional Chinese Medicine.

Wei Qi The defensive energy formed by the lungs.

Wu Xing The Five Elements existing in relationship to each other as seen diagrammatically — typically a five-pointed star enclosed in a circle.

Yin and Yang The philosophy of duality fundamental to Five Element theory.

Zazen From the Japanese Zen tradition (*T'so Ch'an* in Chinese). *Zazen* means 'sitting Zen' and refers to meditation posture, philosophy and practice.

Zen (Chuan in Chinese) A tradition of Buddhism — originating in India — that developed in China and throughout Asia, but is often associated most strongly with Japan. Zen emphasises meditation practice, the beauty of simplicity, discipline and the seeking of one's true nature. Other influences on Japanese Zen include the Mahayana tradition of Buddhism, Confucianism and Daoism. Zen consists of two main schools in Japan, Rinzai and Soto.

Zusanli A *stomach* (Earth) channel point (St.36) in Traditional Chinese Medicine.

Bibliography

Acumoxa Therapy, Volume 1: Reference and Study Guide, Richard Feit and Paul Zmiewski, Paradigm Publications, USA, 1989.

Acupuncture: A Comprehensive Text, Shanghai College of Traditional Medicine (1974), translated and edited by John O'Connor and Dan Bensky, Eastland Press, USA, 1981.

An Outline of Chinese Acupuncture, The Academy of Traditional Chinese Medicine, Foreign Languages Press, Peking (Beijing), China, 1975.

Essentials of Chinese Acupuncture, Foreign Languages Press Beijing, China, 1980.

Healing Ourselves, Naboru Muramoto, Avon Publishing, USA, 1973.

Nan Ching: The Classic of Difficult Issues, Pien Ch'io, translated and annotated by Paul U. Unschild, University of California Press, Calif., 1986.

Nei Ching: The Yellow Emperors Classic of Internal Medicine, translated from the Chinese with introductory study by Ilza Veith, Pelanduk Publications, Malaysia, 1997.

Shiatsu: The Complete Guide, Chris Jarmey and Gabriel Mojay, Thorsons Publishing, UK, 1991.

Tao Te Ching, Lao Tzu, translated by D. C. Lau, Penguin Classics, Penguin Books, UK, 1963.

The Foundations of Chinese Medicine: A Comprehensive Text for Acupuncturists and Herbalists, Giovanni Maciocia, Churchill Livingstone, UK, 1989.

The Web That Has No Weaver: Understanding Chinese Medicine, Ted J. Kaptchuk, Congon & Weed Inc., USA, 1983.

Traditional Acupuncture: Law of the Five Elements, Dianne M. Connelly, The Centre for Traditional Acupuncture, USA, 1979.

Zang Fu Syndromes: Differential Diagnosis and Treatment, John McDonald and Joel Penner, Lone Wolf Press, USA, 1994.

Zen Shiatsu: How to Harmonise Yin and Yang for Better Health, Shizuto Masunaga, Japan Publications Inc., Tokyo and New York, 1977.

Zen Training: Methods and Philosophy, Katsuki Sekida, Weatherhill Publishing, USA, 1975.

Other sources

Many of the ideas and philosophical tenets in this book are adapted from or influenced by translations of works listed in the Bibliography, such as the *Dao Te Ching*. Some of the diagrams and charts are adapted from books, such as *An outline of Chinese Acupuncture,* in the Bibliography above. The origins of commonly held principles and teachings associated with Traditional Chinese Medicine and other philosophies mentioned herein are not always easy to trace and are often handed down from teacher to student or learnt through personal experience. If we have omitted to acknowledge any original work that has contributed to this book we would be happy to hear from you. The following pages contain phrases inspired by the *Dao Te Ching*: 24, 26, 27, 29, 32, 97, 137. The following pages contain text inspired by or drawings and charts adapted from *An outline of Chinese Acupuncture* and *The essentials of Chinese Acupuncture*: 18–22, 25, 39, 48, 65, 73, 89, 96, 110, 118, 135, 140, 159, 174, 175. The following pages contain phrases inspired by the *Nei Ching*: 12, 18–22, 25, 35, 39, 64, 88, 169, 171, 175. Page 99 features a poem from *Zenisms: Laughter on the Path to Enlightenment*, David Bell, Lothian Books, Melbourne, 2002. Page 108 features a poem inspired by Sheng-yen.